CRITI   R

DEATH AND DYING IN
INTENSIVE CARE

FACING DEATH

Series editor: David Clark, Professor of Medical Sociology,
University of Sheffield

The subject of death in late modern culture has become a rich field of theoretical, clinical and policy interest. Widely regarded as a taboo until recent times, death now engages a growing interest among social scientists, practitioners and those responsible for the organization and delivery of human services. Indeed, how we die has become a powerful commentary on how we live and the specialized care of dying people holds an important place within modern health and social care.

This series captures such developments in a collection of volumes which has much to say about death, dying, end of life care and bereavement in contemporary society. Among the contributors are leading experts in death studies, from sociology, anthropology, social psychology, ethics, nursing, medicine and pastoral care. A particular feature of the series is its attention to the developing field of palliative care, viewed from the perspectives of practitioners, planners and policy analysts; here several authors adopt a multi-disciplinary approach, drawing on recent research, policy and organizational commentary, and reviews of evidence-based practice. Written in a clear, accessible style, the entire series will be essential reading for students of death, dying and bereavement and for anyone with an involvement in palliative care research, service delivery or policy making.

Current and forthcoming titles:

David Clark, Jo Hockley and Sam Ahmedzai (eds): *New Themes in Palliative Care*
David Clark and Jane Seymour: *Reflections on Palliative Care*
Mark Cobb: *The Dying Soul: Spiritual Care at the End of Life*
Kirsten Costain Schou and Jenny Hewison: *Experiencing Cancer: Quality of Life in Treatment*
Catherine Exley: *Living with Cancer, Living with Dying*
David Field, David Clark, Jessica Corner and Carol Davis (eds): *Researching Palliative Care*
David Kissane and Sidney Bloch: *Family Grief Therapy*
Gordon Riches and Pam Dawson: *An Intimate Loneliness: Supporting Bereaved Parents and Siblings*
Tony Walter: *On Bereavement: The Culture of Grief*
Jenny Hockey, Jeanne Katz and Neil Small (eds): *Grief, Mourning and Death Ritual*
Jane E. Seymour: *Critical Moments – Death and Dying in Intensive Care*

CRITICAL MOMENTS – DEATH AND DYING IN INTENSIVE CARE

JANE E. SEYMOUR

OPEN UNIVERSITY PRESS
Buckingham • Philadelphia

Open University Press
Celtic Court
22 Ballmoor
Buckingham
MK18 1XW

email: enquiries@openup.co.uk
world wide web: www.openup.co.uk

and
325 Chestnut Street
Philadelphia, PA 19106, USA

First Published 2001

A catalogue record of this book is available from the British Library

ISBN 0 335 20423 6 (pb)   0 335 20424 4 (hb)

Library of Congress Cataloging-in-Publication Data
Seymour, Jane, 1958–
    Critical moments : death and dying in intensive care / Jane E. Seymour.
       p.   cm.
    Includes bibliographical references and index.
    ISBN 0-335-20424-4 – ISBN 0-335-20423-6 (pbk.)
       1. Critical care medicine. 2. Terminal care. 3. Death. 4. Dying. I. Title.

RC86.7.S446 2001
616.029–dc21   00-050496

Typeset by Graphicraft Limited, Hong Kong
Printed in Great Britain by St Edmundsbury Press, Bury St Edmunds, Suffolk

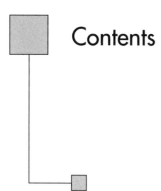

Contents

Series editor's preface

This worthy addition to the Facing Death series denotes a further extension in our range and subject matter. From the outset the series has sought to promote interest in concepts and debates surrounding the phenomenon of human mortality in late modern culture. Several books on the theme of palliative care have appeared (Clark *et al.* 1997, Clark and Seymour 1998, Field *et al.* 2000, Cobb 2001). We have also dealt with some related phenomena in the cancer experience (Costain Schou and Hewison 1998) and in aspects of bereavement (Walter 1999, Riches and Dawson 2000) as well as with the wider cultural dimensions of grief, mourning and death ritual (Hockey *et al.* 2001). Now we have a book which takes us into the heart of the classic modern healthcare institution and the locus of contemporary death, *par excellence*: the hospital. Jane Seymour's brilliant account of the management of critical illness and dying in the setting of the intensive care unit presents new evidence about the way the end of life is shaped, constructed and managed in highly technological healthcare environments. Making use of the ethnographic method it takes us into a world in which doctors, nurses and their colleagues work together first to save lives and where this proves impossible, to then manage the consequences.

In so doing we are given a fascinating view of a modern medical speciality, still striving to consolidate its 'evidence base' and its ethical foundations whilst at the same time further advancing its technical competencies. The rise of intensive care and palliative care follows parallel lines from the late 1950s. Both have become modern, multidisciplinary areas of healthcare specialization, albeit with strikingly different goals in the beginning. If ever two disciplines provided the contrast in orientation between 'care' and 'cure' it might be these. Yet as Jane Seymour shows, intensive care practitioners are often deeply concerned with issues of human dignity, with good communication and with combining skills to provide high quality treatment in ways which are respectful of personhood and bodily integrity. In this sense they have much in common with their colleagues in hospices and specialist palliative care units. Indeed, as we see here, when dealing with dying persons and their companions, intensive care staff, like their palliative care counterparts, are actively engaged in a common purpose: the achievement of 'natural death'. This is fertile ground for sociological analysis. There is something counter-intuitive about the idea that 'hi-tech' healthcare can be compatible with notions of 'nature taking its course'. But if we view all dying as at least in part socially constructed, then the idea begins to resonate.

Such research is a complex terrain for those who engage in it. It presents ethical traps and pitfalls, practical problems of access and acceptance, and requires great personal sensitivity in its conduct. The data so yielded need then to be cracked open and interpreted with skill and insight. In all of these Jane Seymour proves herself more than up to the task. Trained as a social scientist and as a nurse, she also draws upon several years of clinical experience in the intensive care environment. She explains how in approaching her studies she therefore grappled with the roles of both outsider and insider. She writes eloquently and does not shirk dealing with complex biomedical concepts, succeeding in elucidating these for the non-specialist reader. The result is an account which goes beyond the naturalistic naivety of some ethnographic work to produce a rounded and mature analysis of the phenomenon at hand.

Who will benefit from reading such a book? Undoubtedly it will be of interest and create challenges for those already working in intensive care units. It will also appeal to palliative care practitioners whose experience has not extended to the acute healthcare setting. It will certainly interest sociologists, anthropologists and others concerned about the social construction of dying and death, and with questions of inscription, the body and of identity. All of these readers will find in it something of value and insight. *Critical Moments – Death and Dying in Intensive Care* is the work of an accomplished researcher working in a demanding area of study. It will do a great deal to advance understanding of a hitherto little understood area in the sociology of healthcare and I am sure it will be welcomed warmly by readers of the Facing Death series.

References

Clark, D. and Seymour, J. (1998) *Reflections on Palliative Care: Sociological and Policy Perspectives*. Buckingham: Open University Press.
Clark, D., Hockley, J. and Ahmedzai, S. (1997) *New Themes in Palliative Care*. Buckingham: Open University Press.

Cobb, M. (2001) *The Dying Soul: Spiritual Care at the End of Life*. Buckingham: Open University Press.

Costain Schou, K. and Hewison, J. (1998) *Experiencing Cancer: Quality of Life in Treatment*. Buckingham: Open University Press.

Field, D., Clark, D., Corner, J. and Davis, C. (eds) (2000) *Researching Palliative Care*. Buckingham: Open University Press.

Hockey, J., Katz, J. and Small, N. (eds) (2001) *Grief, Mourning and Death Ritual*. Buckingham: Open University Press.

Riches, G. and Dawson, P. (2000) *An Intimate Loneliness: Supporting Bereaved Parents and Siblings*. Buckingham: Open University Press.

Walter, T. (1999) *On Bereavement: The Culture of Grief*. Buckingham: Open University Press.

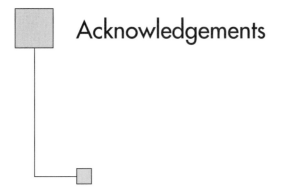

Acknowledgements

The research on which the book is based was supported by a bursary from Trent Palliative Care Centre at the University of Sheffield and was informed by my own work as an intensive care nurse and by many discussions with nursing and medical colleagues during those years. It would not have been possible without the generosity of all the intensive care staff who allowed me to follow their work, and the courage of the patients' families who participated in the study. David Clark was my academic supervisor during three years of doctoral studies: I will always be grateful for his encouragement, support and friendship. My colleagues within the Sheffield Palliative Care Studies Group have also given me invaluable help and support. My family encouraged me to start on this path and have given freely of their love throughout.

Chapter 2 is based on a paper given at an 'Ethnography and Palliative Care' workshop hosted by The Palliative Care Research Forum in London, Cardiff and Edinburgh. It also includes some ideas published in 'Ethical issues in qualitative research at the end of life' published in 1999 (5(2): 65–73) in the *International Journal of Palliative Nursing* and co-authored with Christine Ingleton. Chapter 6 is based on 'Negotiating natural death in intensive care' published by *Social Science and Medicine* in 2000 (51: 1241–52). Chapter 7 expands a paper given in 1997 at the conference of the Critical Care Forum and Royal College of Nursing Research Society 'Developing Practice Through Research: Ideas and Innovations in Critical Care', which was held in Birmingham. Chapter 8 includes material from 'Revisiting medicalization and "natural" death', published in *Social Science and Medicine* in 1999 (49: 691–704).

Notes on fonts, punctuation marks, and use of names and initials

Italics have been used to denote extracts from observational field notes, or to make an emphasis in the text.

... denotes a deleted passage, except where it occurs at the beginning of a quote.

-- denotes a pause in speech.

All names of people and places are pseudonyms. Letters used to denote individuals bear no relevance to their real names.

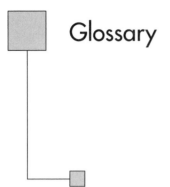

Glossary

This list gives *some* terms which may be unknown to the reader. Others are explained in the text or in notes at the end of chapters.

Drug names have not been included.

AFB	acid-fast bacillus
atrial fibrillation	uncoordinated movement of the atria of the heart
BE	base excess
bradycardia	slow heart rate
cardiomyopathy	disease of the structure and function of the heart
chest creps	breath sounds indicating infection or fluid
CO	cardiac output
creat.	creatinine
CXR	chest X-ray
DC synchronized shock	refers to direct current electrical defibrillation of the heart
GCS	Glasgow Coma Scale
GI	gastro-intestinal
HCO_3	bicarbonate
hemiplegia	one-sided paralysis
hepatic encephalopathy	degenerative brain disorder due to liver disease
hyperglycaemia	high blood glucose
intubation	passage of an endo-tracheal tube for ventilation
IPPV	intermittent positive pressure ventilation
I/V	intravenous
JVP	jugular venous pressure
'micro'	microbiology

NG	naso-gastric
PCO_2	partial pressure of carbon dioxide
PH	potential hydrogen: a scale of acidity of solution
PO_2	partial pressure of oxygen
pulmonary embolism	blood clot in the circulation of the lungs
'RR' or 'rr'	respiratory rate
septic shock	septicaemia induced circulatory collapse marked by multiple organ failure
SIMV	synchronized intermittent mandatory ventilation
SVR	systemic vascular resistance
systolic pressure	systemic blood pressure at the point of ventricular contraction
tachycardia	fast heart rate
tidal volume	size of breath
TPN	intravenous feeding
tracheostomy	creating of access to the trachea via the neck
tricuspid regurgitation	incompetence of a heart valve
'wedge'	indirect measure of left arterial pressure

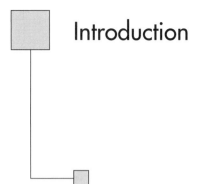

Introduction

The development of the intensive care unit stands as an expression of a post-war medical revolution in which the means have become available to deflect and defer death almost indefinitely. Here, cultural expectations of medical heroism are conjoined with images of the most exacting and precise application of medical science. However, the use of an armoury of scientific and technological advances to try and pull dying people back from the very brink of death has, it might be argued, leapt ahead of our ability to deal with the professional, social, ethical and financial consequences thrown up by its use. Le Fanu (1999: 261), commenting on the 'transforming power' of the technological innovation of artificial ventilation and oxygenation that heralded the development of intensive care in the early 1950s, notes that 50 years later those same life-saving therapies have also become a means of prolonging the 'pain and misery of terminal illness' (1999: 259) for many.

Hospice and palliative care, which developed in its modern form during the same period as intensive care, has gathered a reputation of avoiding overly interventionist treatments and of offering a range of 'low tech' options to people dying with advanced disease (Clark and Seymour 1999). However many people, particularly those suffering from non-cancer conditions that may be less readily labelled as 'terminal', are excluded from its remit. Those who enter the hospital system at a moment of acute illness risk receiving protracted multiple organ support in the hours and days immediately before death. Writing about the use of intensive therapies in American hospitals, Moskowitz and Nelson conjure up a scenario that is increasingly becoming a feature of healthcare provision at the end of life in other parts of the developed world: 'many – perhaps most – Americans now spend their final days surrounded by the technologies of medicine, embedded in a highly specialized, sophisticated setting' (Moskowitz and Nelson 1995: 3).

These risks are highlighted by Paddy Yeoman who, in a personal account of his work as a clinical director of an intensive care unit, recalls the dreadful dilemmas associated with trying to decide whether invasive treatment should be withdrawn from a woman in her mid-seventies. She had undergone dangerous emergency surgery to repair a ruptured aortic aneurysm, and subsequently developed pneumonia and renal failure. She was sedated, placed on a ventilator and given renal dialysis. Days pass during which Dr Yeoman, the surgeon, who had conducted the operation, and the nurses caring for the woman cannot agree on what course of action should be taken. Dr Yeoman and the nurses favour withdrawal of treatment to allow the woman to die peacefully. The surgeon is angry at this suggestion and insists that treatment is continued. The woman's family becomes increasingly distressed and puzzled about what is happening, picking up on the differences of opinion between the intensive care staff and the surgeon. Eventually a compromise is reached, which involves waiting a further 48 hours to see if continued 'full' treatment produces any slight improvement in the woman's condition. Yeoman recalls:

> I suppose you could say that we had struck a deal more than reached a decision. Some could compare it to horse traders haggling for an advantage, or perhaps politicians thrashing out a collective view on a contentious issue . . . For an elderly woman in such a condition it was asking a lot and I felt sure that it was now just a matter of time before we would be stopping treatment and allowing her to die in peace. I didn't hold out much hope, but two days later when I went to her bedside I could see I was wrong. There had been an improvement and what's more, it looked as though it might continue. So we carried on. And she continued to improve, slowly at first and then with a quickening pace . . . she went on to make a complete recovery.
>
> (Yeoman and Sleator 1995: 62)

As this case shows, within intensive care dying and death are not purely technical questions, issues of cost or statistical probability. As Yeoman points out, in this case, recovery was the *least* likely outcome and the cost of treating the patient was huge. She remained in intensive care for eight weeks (at a daily cost of approximately £2000) before she was well enough to be discharged to a general ward. Further, in many other cases of similar severity, actions like these rarely deliver the exceptional recovery experienced by this woman. Such cases prompt accusations of the cruel prolongation of death of otherwise hopelessly ill people and the denial of financial resources to others who could better benefit. Referring to these arguments Yeoman has this to say:

Many would argue that it is an inefficient use of tax-payers' money to spend that amount on one woman in her mid-seventies who in all probability will die within a few years anyway. I can see their point, but they have the luxury of absolute detachment and we have the disadvantage of standing by a patient's bedside where we can see a person rather than a statistic. If that old woman had been their mother, would they hold a different view?

(Yeoman and Sleator 1995: 63)

As these words reveal, issues of non-treatment in intensive care are emotive and, at times, contentious matters which hinge on the resolution of 'problem[s] of social definition' (Glaser and Strauss 1965: 16). This book explores the way in which such resolution occurs and examines the navigation of 'uncertain death at an unknown time' for people who were patients in the intensive care units of two UK city hospitals during the mid-1990s.[1] At the outset, the study was envisaged as an attempt to slow down and dwell on fast-moving action in intensive care in order to better understand the social processes that culminate in a definition of dying and precipitate an application of human agency (in the form of withholding or withdrawing life support) such that death can follow dying.

The 'uncertain/unknown' dying trajectory, identified by Glaser and Strauss (1965) as the least likely route to death during the 1960s, has become not only a fundamental problem attending medical and nursing work at the *bedside* of critically ill people but also a microcosm of *wider* pervasive societal dilemmas regarding end-of-life decision making, the constituents of appropriate care for dying people, and the intersection of ethics, cost containment and technology in the early twenty-first century. An enduring theme throughout this book therefore is an attempt to highlight issues of broad theoretical and clinical interest while representing their 'real' experiential consequences for the individuals involved with dying people in intensive care. The use of case studies and the application of an interpretative approach to the analysis of ethnographic data reflect this overall purpose. Specific 'critical incidents' occurring during fieldwork are used to illuminate issues of more general applicability. In the chapters that follow, we join critically ill people and their attendants on a journey through uncertainty: from the early days of admission to intensive care to death or recovery. The research on which the book is based consisted of 14 case studies completed in the intensive care units of two large hospitals in the UK.

Chapter 1 sets the scene for the empirical chapters that follow by examining the short history of intensive care and exploring a range of issues associated with its provision. I spend some time making comparisons between intensive care units in the UK and the US, before turning to an exploration of the insights that may be gleaned from earlier ethnographies about illness, dying and death in acute hospital environments and a discussion of the extent to which dying in hospital has been characterized as a threat to 'good death'. Chapter 2 is a personal account of conducting ethnography within the highly charged setting of intensive care in which I draw together some reflections and thoughts about the ethical issues I encountered during the fieldwork period. Chapters 3–8 have a central theme running throughout: the treatment of decision making as a social process bounded by particular organizational contexts, rather than a product of individual reasoning governed by immutable ethical and scientific principles. In the analysis of these interrelated issues these empirical chapters bring together three themes in contemporary sociological theory and relate them to traditional issues of nursing concern.

First, I employ insights from the social constructionist perspective on medical knowledge to examine how clinical data informing prognosis are assembled, read, and interpreted during clinical work. Medical staff are the primary focus of this examination. Intensive care offers a particularly rich opportunity to examine the utility of this perspective, for not only is intensive care medicine complex, concentrated and interspecialized, but it is also conducted around a 'patient' who, by virtue of the severity of his or her condition, cannot interact in the everyday, taken for granted sense of the word.

Second, I locate this analysis of medicine in the context of its co-existence with nursing. In the available literature, this co-existence is portrayed as beset with problems. These concern the differential location of nurses and doctors on a 'cure–care' continuum, the relatively powerless position of nursing in relation to medicine, as well as dysfunctional patterns of 'coping' during nurses' interactions with dying patients and their companions. The concept of a 'negotiated order' (Strauss 1979; Svensson 1996) is employed to interpret the close and symbiotic nature of the relationship between medicine and nursing in intensive care. This enables the book to move beyond a position which suggests that nursing and medicine exist in a viewpoint of polarized opposition, and allows instead an analysis of their 'shared' situation.

Third, I use insights from contemporary debates about the meaning, formation and retrospective construction of 'good death' to analyse the experiential accounts given by patients' companions. In this analysis a major concern is to elicit those features of healthcare practice that respondents perceive as supportive of 'good death'; and to engender some sense of the interpenetration of individual emotional experience with the conduct of clinical work.

Chapter 3 examines the early phase of critical illness, shortly after admission to intensive care, and focuses on the way in which diagnostic uncertainty is resolved during medical work. Chapter 4 focuses closely on the intersection between medical and nursing work in intensive care, while Chapter 5 turns to an exploration of the extent to which patients' companions are involved in the process of care planning. The emphasis here is on the disclosure of information to companions and the various ways in which they use and interpret such information. Chapters 6 and 7 examine the processes that underpin the withdrawal of active medical treatment, and explore the movement to 'nursing care only' for dying people. The social construction of 'natural death' during clinical work is explored in these chapters. Chapter 8 examines the narrative reconstruction of events in intensive care by patients' companions and presents a conceptual reformulation of 'good death'.

In Chapter 9, the main themes of previous chapters are drawn together and their implications for healthcare practice are explored.

The research on which this book is based had its origins in my work as a nurse in intensive care units in the UK between 1984 and 1994, although the observations, documentary analyses and interviews comprising the case studies were carried out during 1995 and the first few months of 1996. Clearly, the experience of working in intensive care as a nurse and the business of conducting ethnography in the same environment are, to some extent, indissoluble: the first led to the second, and will have had a major impact on the questions I posed and on the way in which I interpreted what I saw, heard, and reported the latter. Indeed, one of the units in which I had worked for four years was chosen as the first research setting. The second setting was a completely unfamiliar unit. Making this choice was partly pragmatic, insofar as it was much easier to gain access where I was a known and trusted individual; and partly related to my belief that any unforeseen ethical problems associated with the actual conduct of the research would be best 'ironed out' somewhere where staff were likely to be honest and truthful, rather than polite, with me.

My practical experience as a nurse and my academic background as a sociologist means that nursing and sociological approaches intersect within the book. I hope that each 'view' has enriched the other in a rather unusual and insightful way. In effect, each perspective stands here as a potential critique of the other, allowing each to enter territories not usually 'seen' or acknowledged as important in research placed within one discipline. The risk in a project like this is, however, that certain questions will not be answered to the satisfaction of different sections of the readership. This is probably inevitable, but it is hoped that the detailed presentation of data in the subsequent chapters will allow readers to draw their own conclusions as to the worth of the interpretation presented.

Note

1 Glaser and Strauss (1965: 16) describe four 'types' of death expectation:

    1 certain death at a known time;
    2 certain death at an unknown time;

3 uncertain death, but a known time when the question will be resolved;
4 uncertain death and unknown time when the question will be resolved.

Glaser and Strauss's analysis of awareness contexts focused on the first three types of death expectation. It might be suggested that the fourth type is now a central concern in high-technology healthcare practice.

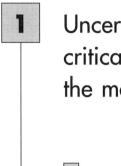

1 Uncertain deaths: critical care and the modern hospital

This chapter is organized into three sections. The first gives an account of the history of intensive care, its intersection with the modern hospital, and the range of issues with which it contends. The second identifies insights from sociological studies concerned with the construction, negotiation, definition and management of illness and death, and draws on studies relating specifically to intensive care and other acute areas of the hospital organization. The third section examines the extent to which the experience and nature of death in hospitals has been characterized as a threat to 'good death'.

Intensive care: history and relationship with the modern hospital

Intensive care developed primarily in the post second world war period in order to provide medical and nursing care to seriously ill individuals with potentially curable conditions. Its emergence coincided with the development of techniques of artificial ventilation, of cardio-pulmonary resuscitation and of increasingly complex surgical and medical procedures. A particular influence was the realization in Denmark during the polio epidemic of 1948–1953 that intermittent positive pressure ventilation,[1] using a cuffed tracheostomy tube and a manually inflated rubber bag on an anaesthetized patient, was an effective treatment for bulbar poliomyelitis (Ambiavagar and McConn 1978). Gilbertson (1995) points out that this revolutionary new method of treating respiratory failure 'opened the theatre doors to anaesthetists by giving them a new role in the care of the critically ill, and has been considered to have marked the beginning of intensive therapy' (Gilbertson 1995: 459p). Such a method replaced the awful, and usually hopeless techniques, of trying to introduce air into the lungs of an awake agonized dying person using a facemask or by applying pressure to either side of the rib cage. Moreover, the new method was more flexible, less clumsy and more mobile to use than the giant 'iron lung'[2] tanks used previously to treat the victims of chronic respiratory failure.

The movement of anaesthetic specialists out of the operating room and into post-operative 'recovery' areas further influenced the growth of intensive care. Their expertise allowed for the development of biochemical, haematological and physiological monitoring to an unprecedented extent. This, together with the availability of new drugs and techniques to treat multiple organ failure and sepsis, constituted the 'technologies of rescue' (Reiser 1992) that were the catalyst for the exponential growth of intensive care.

There is some dispute about where the very first intensive care unit opened, although Schechter *et al.* (1998) argue convincingly that it was the 'special intensive care unit' opened by Dr J. Murray Beardsley in Rhode Island in 1955. Beardsley, writing in 1956 about the care of seriously ill surgical patients, argued that 'the more efficient approach to the problem is to segregate all seriously ill patients in a single unit that is staffed by personnel especially trained for the job' (Schechter *et al.* 1998: 318). Under his direction a new 28-bedded unit opened to receive patients straight from the nearby operating theatre.

The US witnessed a much more rapid, and early, expansion of intensive care than that seen in the UK. The mechanism of hospital payment in the US drove forward this expansion; since the prevailing method of insurance reimbursement allowed hospitals to gather payments *after* expensive treatments had been given. For this reason, hospitals across the country were able to purchase the latest technologies and charge them off as part of the costs of care (Reiser 1992). Developments in post-operative care, which allowed complex cardiac surgery to be performed successfully, are just one notable example of a range of techniques that were quickly adopted as part of the intensive care armoury.

The especially rapid adoption of 'technologies of rescue' (Reiser 1992) in the US means that the character of 'intensive care' in that country differs somewhat from that in the UK. The first and most obvious difference is that units in the US tend to be much larger than those in the UK. As in the Rhode Island example, units of 20 or more beds are not uncommon in the US, while in the UK units tend to be much smaller, sometimes containing only four or five beds. Similarly, intensive care units are much more evenly spread across all areas of the US. In the UK, the availability of intensive care is unevenly spread across the country (Metcalfe and McPherson 1994; Audit Commission 1999), although it is an accepted principle that all hospitals have access to some form of intensive care facility. Overall, in the UK, only 1 per cent of beds in the acute sector are in intensive care (2 per cent when speciality specific units are included) but the number of such beds is increasing rapidly. Nine out of 10 acute NHS Trusts now have some form of intensive care unit, and many have coronary care, high dependency and speciality specific units as well (Audit Commission 1999). Baldock (1995), commenting on the expansion in demand for intensive care beds in the UK, suggests that this has resulted from a steady growth in emergency admissions to hospital accompanied, paradoxically, by a decline in the availability of non-intensive care acute beds (Metcalfe and McPherson 1994; D. Bennett 1995).

A second major difference between the UK and the US intensive care units concerns the character of the patient caseload. In the US the clinical caseload shows more variation than that in the UK, with a tendency to admit patients who are either far more, or far less ill than would be the case in the UK. In contrast in the UK, a picture has been drawn in both the medical and national press of 'inappropriate admissions', that is, people who either are too well or too ill to benefit from intensive care. Fuelling this latter portrayal have been anecdotes of individual patients who were refused admission, and reports of scarcity of beds meaning that 'appropriate patients' have to be transported between hospitals in a desperate search for beds (Metcalfe *et al.* 1997).

The SUPPORT study (Principal Investigators for the SUPPORT Project 1995) is one of the biggest sources of evidence about the trend of admitting very ill patients to intensive care in the US, showing that 38 per cent of hospitalized patients who die as a result of life-threatening illness spend at least 10 days in intensive care immediately preceding death, even in those cases where a 'do not resuscitate' order has been written. Further evidence of this tendency may be gleaned from an observational study of hospital deaths conducted in the US during the early 1990s by Kaufman (1998). Of the 80 deaths that Kaufman observed among older adults in one American hospital over a 12-month period, 31 occurred in intensive care. Figures for the total number of deaths for adults over 50, which occurred at that hospital during the observational period, showed that out of 370 deaths, one-third took place in intensive care. Commenting on why there is such a preponderance of dying people in intensive care units in the US, Kaufman (1998: 724) notes that 'the diffuse power of litigation that hangs over every hospital activity' has contrived to make the recognition of dying and the cessation of acute interventionist treatment a nigh impossibility in the US.

This differential growth of intensive care in the US and the UK is exemplified in the timing of the recognition of a distinct sub-speciality of clinical medicine in each country. In the UK, this did not occur until 1987, although it must be noted that the proposal had been mooted as early as 1967 (Hunter 1967). In the US a Society of Critical Care Medicine was founded years earlier in 1970 (Parrillo 1995).

One of the most distinctive characteristics of modern intensive care across the developed world is the central role played by nursing staff. In the UK, units are staffed traditionally according to a 1:1 nurse:patient ratio, while in the US the ratio is more variable. This probably reflects, as noted above, the greater range in severity of illness of patients admitted to intensive care in the US. Nurses employed in such units have an extensive specialist training and relative autonomy in a forum of work that appears to be predominantly medical-technical in orientation (Walby and Greenwell 1994). Thus, intensive care nurses work alongside medical staff in an unusually close, and often interchangeable, way. It has been acknowledged that many intensive care nurses have a status *vis à vis* medicine that is almost unparalleled. The source of such status would appear to be their 'medical' orientation and proficient use of highly technological machinery (Lynaugh and Fairman 1992).

In many ways, 'intensive care' represents, in a symbolic and real sense, the modern preoccupation with the mastery of disease, the eradication of 'untimely death' and the prolongation of life. It is the place to which clinicians may refer a patient when that individual stands at the brink of death and is beyond the reach of conventional therapies. It has become a necessary and routine part of the post-operative management of some increasingly complex surgical procedures (Crosby and Rees 1994). It has even begun to play a role in the palliative management of patients suffering from conditions such as AIDS and invasive cancer (Schapira *et al.* 1993; Gelder 1995), particularly haematological malignancies. Further, a spill-over effect can be observed, with treatments once limited to intensive care units becoming incorporated into 'ordinary' practice within the hospital organization, and thus becoming part of the expected range of available interventions directed at achieving 'cure' or deferral of death in almost all circumstances of illness.[3] The development of high dependency units, of coronary care units, of specialist units for the treatment of renal, liver or neurosurgical conditions are clear examples of this trend (Thompson and Singer 1995; Audit Commission 1999).

The trend of patient admission to adult intensive care units tends to reflect both demographic patterns and the hospital population as a whole. Thus, a growing proportion of intensive care patients are elderly and suffering from an acute exacerbation of a long-term chronic illness rather than from the effects of infectious disease or sudden trauma (Dragsted and Qvist 1992). While case mix varies between units, the tensions (which are perhaps a defining feature of modern hospital care) caused by financial constraints, demography and technology are captured in a particularly acute way within intensive care. Here, patients who once would have died quickly from their conditions may now recover. However, as yet this is an unpredictable outcome. Of those patients admitted to intensive care, between 15 and 35 per cent die during intensive therapy (Koch *et al.* 1994; Metcalfe and McPherson 1994; Audit Commission 1999), and others die shortly after discharge. Ridley *et al.* (1990) studied the outcome of 497 patients admitted to their UK intensive care unit over a two-year period. Forty-eight per cent of all patients died within two years, with death being particularly common for patients over the age of 65, of whom 53 per cent died within two years. More recently, in the UK the Audit Commission (1999: 22) estimates that 37 per cent of all patients admitted to intensive care units die within six months; a figure that varies with unit case mix and also, possibly, with clinical approach:

> Given that survival rates vary between units even when patient differences are taken into account, the likelihood is that differences in clinical approach also affect survival. Such differences could be due to many things, ranging from individual choice of approach through to the amount of time available for each patient or the equipment or drugs available for use
>
> (Audit Commission 1999: 23)

In the US 1 per cent of the domestic gross national product is spent annually on intensive care (Jennett 1994), while in the UK available estimates suggest that the costs of intensive therapy is up to six times as great as treatment on general wards. The Audit Commission (1999) estimates that the UK annual bill for intensive care is £675–725 million, and is increasing at 5 per cent per year. Commenting on the 'modern epidemic' of multiple organ failure, Bion and Strunin observe that many of the costs come from the administration of supportive techniques for multiple organ failure.[4]

> ... it costs twice as much to die in an intensive care unit as it does to survive [and] the resources to generate a survivor are considerable. For those patients destined to die, prognostic uncertainty encourages protracted organ system support, with the result that death is merely deferred at greater expense.
>
> (Bion and Strunin 1996: 1)

Recognition of this situation has led to a growing concern among intensive care clinicians to develop individual indicators of prognosis (Knaus *et al.* 1991; Atkinson *et al.* 1994; Gunning and Rowan 1999) and to an extensive debate about the rationing of intensive therapy (Bion 1995). This latter debate, which has focused particularly on the utility of age as a means of determining a level of treatment provision (Baltz and Wilson 1995), has developed alongside a parallel debate about the most appropriate ways of stopping the delivery of 'futile' treatments. The debate about the ethics of advance directives (Doyal 1995), the differences between active and passive euthanasia and physician-assisted suicide (Pappas 1996), all bear witness to the complex intersection between clinical medicine and ethics that now attend the delivery, rationing and withdrawal of high-technology treatments.

Moreover, ethical principles have been revealed to be in a state of flux. As Singer notes in his commentary on the changing and historically situated nature of medical ethics:

when it comes to questions about prolonging life or ending it, our ethics are in a confused contradictory mess . . . The advances of medical technology have forced us to think about issues that we previously had no need to face . . . Technology creates an imperative: 'If we can do it, we will do it.' Ethics asks: 'We can do it, but should we do it?' But the ethic within which we try to answer this question stands on shaky foundations that few of us now accept. Confused and contradictory judgements are the result.

(Singer 1994: 17–19)

Singer's analysis of the confusion in medical ethics points to the variety of interpretations that can be placed on what were once seemingly incontrovertible and clear 'moments' of transition between life and death. The concept of 'brain death' has superseded earlier definitions of death, but as Singer notes, this has led to an extensive debate about the nature and meaning of human consciousness. Drawing on an analysis of the legal arguments surrounding the Tony Bland case (*Airedale NHS Trust* v *Bland* 1993), he demonstrates the range of interpretations that are now possible regarding the very basis of 'meaningful' life and the slippery distinctions between allowing timely death and procuring untimely death.

Recognition of the ethical and diagnostic complexity surrounding death has led to a trend in medicine to search for ever greater precision in the *technical* specification of disease, thus developing a 'science of prognosis' (Searle 1996: 291). This, together with a search for practical 'guidelines' with which to negotiate ethical dilemmas, has resulted in a move towards the removal of 'private' clinical judgement and its replacement with 'public', accountable, and 'evidence'-based practice. The move towards clinical governance is a clear example of this trend, demanding that intensive care units make publicly available not only the outcomes of their care, but also the decision-making processes that lead to those outcomes. The Audit Commission (1999), in a candid discussion of the difficulties that lie behind such 'new ground', poses a number of questions that need to be considered if this move towards 'transparency' is meaningful. For example, in raising the issue of 'futility', it asks: 'can there be a central definition of what constitutes "futile surgery" . . . Or should it be left to individual trusts aided perhaps by scoring systems that can estimate the likely extent of post-operative care needed for a patient?' (Audit Commission 1999: 90).

Turner's insight into the impact of medical-technological advances on the division between life and death, and the sequelae for end-of-life care, captures the difficulty of prioritizing 'technical' indices over and above the more elusive, but no less critical, socially constructed criteria produced during team interaction:

the problem, however, is not simply technical since there is an essential difference between medical death and social death. Dying is a social process, involving changes in behaviour and a process of assessment which do not necessarily correspond to the physical process of bodily death. Death, like birth, has to be socially organized and, in the modern hospital, is an outcome of team activities

(Turner 1996: 198)

This insight into the social nature and organization of death emerged originally as a result of observational studies conducted during the 1960s. These prompted an interest into the way in which the 'problem' of death was managed during social interaction. Later studies explored the differential distribution of knowledge, cognition (Schutz 1964; Cicourel 1974, 1990) and power between professionals involved in such interactions. The emergence of social constructionism in medical sociology (Bury 1986; Nicholson and McLaughlin 1987, 1988) allowed for a refinement of such ideas, which suggested that the ways in which 'dying' became known and recognized was not merely an issue of the *distribution* or allocation of knowledge to various parties in the interaction, but involved the active construction of that knowledge during group interaction, conversation, and routine practices. In this latter perspective the dying patient almost disappears as a material entity, to re-emerge in a socially reproduced form.

A major theme in this book is an examination of the social construction of dying during the clinical work of medicine and nursing. Both disciplines will be portrayed as occupying a shared situation in which, although their 'work' is defined discursively, they are sometimes able to negotiate shared solutions to the management of dying and death within an overwhelmingly curative environment. An attempt has been made to portray the people who occupy nursing and medical roles as thinking, feeling, emotionally embodied selves who communicate on several levels, both formal and informal, lay and professional. The next section of this chapter turns to how such issues have been conceptualized in earlier sociological analyses.

Sociological analyses of illness, dying and death in acute hospital environments

Glaser and Strauss (1965) described the interactions between staff and patients in six hospitals in San Francisco. Their seminal study was a pivotal influence in the development of research looking at the care and management of dying people in hospital environments. They introduced the concept of 'awareness': 'who, in the dying situation, knows what about the probabilities of death for the dying patient' (1965: ix). The primary focus of their analysis was on the types of social action engaged in by healthcare staff to avoid direct disclosure of a poor prognosis and how this led to the isolation of dying persons and those close to them. Sudnow (1967) was similarly concerned with the social action surrounding the dying. He argued that dying places a 'frame of interpretation' around people resulting in 'social death' practices that serve to isolate them. Sudnow, and Glaser and Strauss, detailed strategies employed by hospital staff to cope with the threat of death. Glaser and Strauss were particularly concerned with the relationship between nurses, doctors and their patients, analysing the sequelae that flow from the unpredictability of 'slow dying' trajectories within hospitals. They described the way in which nurses and doctors would practise avoidance of death by means of pretence in the delivery of information and by attention to routine tasks. They suggested that such practices would persist until such time as 'dying' became the subject of 'open awareness' for all parties.

These ideas are related to those developed by Goffman (1968, 1974), in his analysis of the interactional formation of identity in institutions, and by Perakyla (1991). Perakyla applied the concept of 'frame' to an analysis of the way in which hospital staff achieve, through interaction, a transformation of 'curative' hope to palliative 'hope' within hospital wards. He showed how, as the hope that patients will be cured diminishes, a skilful slanting in conversation achieves a different emphasis. The patient thus becomes someone who will 'feel better' even though they may not 'get better' (1991: 420).

The above studies used insights from symbolic interactionist theory to introduce the idea that death was not a moment that could be recognized irrefutably, but rather that death, the process of dying, and the meanings with which it was associated were a product of social interaction. In this conceptualization, dying is fashioned by organizational contexts and by the particular patterns of social conduct within those organizations. Sudnow outlined his theoretical perspective thus: 'the categories of hospital life, e.g. "life", "illness", "patient", "dying", "death" or whatever are to be seen as constituted by practices of hospital personnel as they engage in their daily routinized interactions within an organizational milieu' (Sudnow 1967: 8). Sudnow concluded that dying was socially defined by hospital personnel to the extent that the actual moment of biological death became dissociated temporally from the moment of 'social death'; that is, the point at which an individual was treated as if biological death has already occurred. In the usual pattern of events, patients who approach death may be subjected to pre-death treatment, which confirms their status as non-persons. Sudnow describes how bodies of still living, but comatose, patients would be partially prepared for the morgue, or would be removed to spatially separate areas away from the main wards. Further, such dissociation between social and biological death was not, in Sudnow's observations, uni-directional. A clear example Sudnow gives in which social death does not occur until *after* biological death is the arrival of a biologically dead person in casualty, whose family are told that 'everything is being done' to save them. A time period elapses before staff go and tell the family that death has occurred.

This time lapse allows 'death to be seen as the outcome of dying' (1967: 95), and reduces the potential threat which such sudden and unexpected death may pose to social and sentimental order. Sudnow demonstrated that such practices were influenced very directly by the perceived social worth of individual patients.

While some have questioned the applicability of Sudnow's observations of the 1960s to the situation some 40 years later (see, for example, Bauman 1992), a recently published ethnography of the use of cardio-pulmonary resuscitation (CPR) in the emergency departments of two US hospitals suggests that they are highly relevant to the current scene. In his account of the manner in which medical and nursing staff 'manage' CPR, Timmermans notes that:

> certain outstanding social characteristics have significant moral connotations that affect the intensity with which the staff approaches the resuscitative effort. The most outstanding social characteristics are age and the perceived seriousness of the illness. These variables, of course have medical meanings, but the strong value judgements about the patient's quality of life – present and future – attached to age and perceived seriousness of illness render these variables social.
>
> (Timmermans 1999: 124)

Zussman's (1992) ethnography of two intensive care units in the US suggests that nursing and medicine occupy diametrically opposed positions along the care–cure continuum which leads to conflict and confusion over the dying process, and a different stance over the pursuit of 'heroic' activities such as CPR. In a stark characterization of the apparent powerlessness of nursing discourse to influence patient care, Zussman observes that: 'nurses may concern themselves with care rather than cure, with the social and emotional aspects of illness rather than the physiology, but in the ICU they are rarely able to express that concern . . . they are not "angels of mercy". Like physicians, they have become technicians' (Zussman 1992: 80).

In a study of neo-natal intensive care, Anspach (1987, 1988, 1993) characterizes the relationship between nurses and physicians as being essentially conflictual. She develops ideas from Freidson's (1970) analysis of the social application of medical knowledge, arguing that the socially organized division of labour between the two professions structures the way in which they perceive the prognosis of sick babies in their care. Knowledge becomes differentially distributed between the two groups, with doctors relying on diagnostic technology as an 'interpretative lens' (Anspach 1987: 215) through which to view prognosis and nurses relying on interactive and perceptual cues.

Anspach's observations are supported by Slomka (1992), who portrays how doctors, nurses and families bring different interpretations and perceptions to the condition of the dying patient in intensive care. These have to be 'bargained' for or 'negotiated' in a situation of unequal power:

> bargaining for, or negotiating reality is a process in which actors each
> with a different view of what is true about a situation attempt to make
> their view of the situation prevail . . . success in the negotiation will
> depend on the position of relative power [that] each person can claim
> in the context
>
> (Slomka 1992: 252)

From a nursing and sociological perspective, Degner and Beaton (1987) conducted a four-year study examining 'life and death decisions' in Canadian hospitals, looking in some detail at intensive care units. They described patterns of control in decision making and the type of prognostic 'calculations' made by individual participants during treatment deliberations. Accounting for the frequent problems of nurse–doctor disagreement in such situations, Degner and Beaton (1987: 56) note that: 'nurses and physicians differ in their getting better-getting worse calculations. Such differences of opinion are common between physicians and nurses, and are usually related to their use of different criteria.'

Zussman, Anspach, Slomka and Degner and Beaton all portray power and knowledge in a similar way. In their analyses, power is 'held' differentially by various groups in the intensive care environment, and is exercised consciously in the form of particular strategies and tactics in order to maintain influence and control over the treatment and care of patients. Nursing and medicine, in these characterizations and others (Field 1989; Walby and Greenwell 1994; MacKay 1993), are unitary 'world views' to which individuals ascribe through professional socialization. In a conceptualization, which has become widely accepted as legitimate, nursing and medicine are merely different, separately constituted, and more or less powerful perspectives on a *given* subject.

Several theorizations are available which suggest that such analyses may be questioned. Svensson (1996) for example, draws on analyses of the doctor–nurse game (Stein 1967; Hughes 1988; Stein *et al.* 1990) to point out that there may be an informal, not readily recognizable, slippage of power between the two professions. He combines this observation with the concept of a negotiated social order (Strauss 1979). Svensson suggests that as the social contexts found in hospitals become ever more complex and less subject to definitive policies and rules, then 'space' is created for interpretation and negotiation of the possible, the legitimate and the appropriate (1996: 381). These do not always involve observable power relations as Slomka (1992) implies. Svensson (1996) develops these insights to suggest on the basis of his research that the very concepts with which medicine and nursing operate become constructed through their day-to-day interactions with each other. Here, rather than a potentially destructive collision between two opposed standpoints, there is a constant negotiation and re-negotiation of that which medicine and nursing *actually consist*. More fundamentally, some analysts follow Foucault (1976) and suggest that the clinical subject of nursing and medicine, the patient's body, is actively constructed through medical and nursing discourse:

> a Foucauldian perspective . . . contends that there is no such thing as an authentic human body that exists outside medical practice and medical discourse. Rather, the body and its various parts are understood as constructed through discourses and practices, through the 'clinical gaze' exerted by practitioners
>
> (Lupton 1997: 99)

In this perspective, professional power is disguised, complex and creative. It flows between professional groups and individuals, depending on collusion and persuasion. Rather than the domination of one professional group by another, there is a diffusion of ideas in which certain modes of description become accepted as rational, scientific and credible bases for action. Arney and Bergen's observation of the insidious nature of medical power over attitudes to death makes the point clearly: 'today we cannot think about death except in a language informed by medicine' (1984: 37).

Most analyses that have employed insights from this perspective in the hospital context have focused on the doctor–patient interaction (Strong 1979; Fisher 1984; Silverman 1987), the nurse–patient interaction (Armstrong 1983b, May 1992a,b), or have looked at the discourse that takes place between doctors (Muller and Koenig 1988; Fox 1992; Atkinson 1995). Sociological and anthropological research that influenced these recent analyses of clinical work in high-technology areas of medicine tends similarly to focus on doctor–doctor interaction (Crane 1975; Millman 1976; Bosk 1979; Eisenberg 1979; Katz 1985; Clark *et al.* 1991). These studies drew attention to the prevalence of 'non medical' criteria in medical decision making, illustrating Freidson's observation that diagnosis and treatment are not: 'biological acts common to mice, monkeys and men' (1970: 209) but are socially determined and structured choices.

One of the earliest studies of this kind was that conducted by Fox (1959) in a clinic for the treatment of and research into metabolic disorders. Fox examined the role of uncertainty in medical practice, highlighting that medicine in an era of high technology is faced with a huge range of diagnostic choices and disposal possibilities. Following Fox, other commentators began to look at the way in which doctors learn, during the course of professional socialization, to manage uncertainty in the course of medical practice (Knafl and Burkett 1975; Atkinson 1981, 1984). Studies such as those by Atkinson (1992), Bloor (1976, 1978a,b, 1994) and Berg (1992) suggest that habitual patterns of behaviour are used to manage variations met during clinical practice. Thus, during the various meetings, ward rounds and record-keeping activities that constitute medical work, standard routines are employed to respond to clinical problems. In this way, medicine becomes a paradigm (Berg 1992: 171) which pre-structures exactly what it is that the doctor *sees* in front of him- or herself.

In some sense, the analysts above make a collectively persuasive case for an image of medicine as a discursive prison. Within the confines of this prison, some slight movement is possible, but that movement is strictly controlled in terms of its latitude or flexibility of response. Here, dying and death must be accommodated within those same discursive routines and rules. It may be hypothesized on the basis of such a conceptualization, therefore, that where death and dying occur in the intensive care environment (where curative treatment is the *raison d'être*) then they will not necessarily be perceived as anything more than an *acute* episode of illness, with a series of approved methods of treatment.

Some commentators suggest however, that such analyses rely on the 'official' version of medical encounters and do not pay adequate attention to the possibility of *resistance* to predominant discourses or to the intricacies of the interpersonal encounters that take place during clinical work (Lupton 1997). Available accounts that do focus on resistance, explore the relationship between patients and healthcare staff. Bloor and McIntosh (1990), for example, report the various strategies employed by mothers to avoid the surveillance of health visitors. However, analyses that focus on the resistance of clinical practitioners (either solely or in conjunction with others) to mainstream discourses are lacking. Lupton's observation may be pertinent to an understanding of the relationships that are enacted during the course of clinical work:

[there may be] different sources of self [which] intertwine and become important at different times for the same person. In this conceptualisation, subjectivity may be understood as dynamic and contextual rather than static, and as often fraught with ambivalence, irrationality and conflict. It is this recognition of the continual ambivalence of subjectivity that may provide some insights into the ways that people are often complicit in the reproduction of medical power as well as frequently seeking to challenge it.

(Lupton 1997: 106)

This book characterizes the enactment of medicine as a publicly oriented job of work, performed by individuals who may employ alternative discursive frameworks in their day-to-day dealings with critically ill and dying patients. Such alternative frameworks are employed very frequently during their exchanges with nurses, usually in recognition of nurses' more psychosocial orientation towards dying patients and their companions. It can be argued that nurses' psychosocial and 'private' view of the patient has been influenced by ideas from the 'good death' movement exemplified by hospice and palliative care. This latter movement developed largely in response to, and as a rejection of, culturally held images of hospitalized death as the archetypal 'bad death'. The next section of the chapter will examine the ways in which death in hospital has been characterized in this literature.

Dying in hospital: a threat to 'good death?'

> While it is true that seriously ill people generally seek out hospitals in the hope of staving off death, it is also true that the anticipation of 'hospitalised death' can be accompanied by a special kind of fear: that the dying will be caught up in a medical juggernaut driven by a logic of its own, one less focused on human suffering and dignity than on the struggle to maintain vital functions.
>
> (Moskowitz and Nelson 1995)

In this statement Moskowitz and Nelson, who are commenting on the SUPPORT study (Principal Investigators for the SUPPORT Project 1995), betray the paradoxical attitudes towards modern illness, treatment and death that have emerged partly in response to the difficulties associated with the definition and management of death in hospitals. Some insight into these ambiguous tensions can be obtained by an exploration of the influences that contribute both to societal attitudes towards death and dying, and to the rhetoric of healthcare practice with dying people.

The growth of the modern hospital has been a defining feature of twentieth-century health care. Within its environs, most of us are born and many later receive treatment for a huge and bewildering variety of medical problems. However, the most salient feature of the hospital is, perhaps, the way in which it has assumed the care of dying people together with the control and definition of the very process of dying. Hospitals have now not only become the place of death for the majority of people (Griffin 1991) but are also the environment in which an increasing proportion of the last year of life is spent. Data from a survey conducted in the UK by Seale and Cartwright (1994) show that people who died during 1986 spent an average of 38 days in hospitals or hospices in the year before their death. This figure represents 22 per cent of all occupied NHS bed days during that year (Seale and Cartwright 1994: 127).

It can be argued that much of the literature and research concerning the modern 'way' and attitude to death contains a common, pervasive theme. In essence, this theme is that of a critique of hospitalized, medicalized death and its representation as a threat to an idealized 'good death'. Hospitalized death, in this literature, is characterized by a loss of individual choice, fear, isolation from family, friends and professional carers, lack of knowledge about the dying state and by a prolongation of the dying career. Lofland (1978) identified six defining features of contemporary death, which combine powerfully to produce these experiences:

1 a high level of medical technology;
2 early disease detection;
3 a complex definition of death;
4 a high prevalence of chronic disease;
5 a low incidence of fatal injuries;
6 active intervention in the dying process.

One of the most powerful influences on contemporary literature associated with death and dying has been Ariès's (1976, 1981) historical descriptions of those events. In what has been called a 'romantic' account of a 'bad present in the name of a better past' (Elias 1985: 12), Ariès presents a compelling and convincing 'grand narrative' of the loss of the 'simple familiarity' (Ariès 1981: 18) of 'tame' death and its eventual replacement by the 'dirty' and 'wild' event of medicalized death. Here, dying and death are redefined as technical problems, managed within the confines of the hospital by medical experts and enveloped in unpredictability and medical mystery. The processes, trajectory and very definition of dying become uncertain, divorced from 'lay' understanding, and culturally and religiously barren. Drawing inspiration from Illich's analysis of 'medical nemesis', in which Illich argues that modern medicine has 'brought the epoch of natural death to an end' (1976: 210), Ariès concludes by positing the image of medicalized death as the icon of the 'bad' death: 'The death of the patient in hospital, covered with tubes, is becoming a more popular image than the *transi* or skeleton of macabre rhetoric' (1981: 614).

Lending credence to this powerful image have been empirical studies of the problems of social isolation associated with the management of dying in the curative environment of acute hospitals (Glaser and Strauss 1965; Quint 1967; Sudnow 1967; McIntosh 1977; Bond 1983; Field 1989; Wilkinson 1991); together with enduring concerns associated with the availability of new technologies that can blur the boundaries between living and dying. Kastenbaum's description of 'phenomenological death' (1969), where dying people exist under sedation and trapped in an isolated state of suspended animation, perhaps best captures the image of death most feared under high-technology medical care. Here, advanced technology is conceptualized as a 'driving force' (Moller 1990: 37), which leads inexorably to the isolation of the dying person and the dehumanization of death. As Timmermans notes (1998: 148), 'the observation that it is impossible for advanced medical technology and humane, dignified dying to co-exist becomes thus both an assumption and a normative conclusion'.

One particularly influential response to the demise of the 'good' death has been the hospice and palliative care movement. Hospice and palliative care has developed an ideology of personal knowledge, control and choice, conjoined with control of physical suffering by the judicious use of (preferably) 'low' technology clinical interventions (Field 1994, 1996) in which the 'natural' course of dying is reclaimed from the threat of the vice-like grip of more advanced 'high' technology clinical interventions. The persuasiveness of the hospice 'way' of death lies perhaps in its promise to bring to fruition an image of late modern 'good' death, as described by Elias (1985): in bed, at home and under benign medical care in which interventions to ensure painlessness are balanced with the autonomous choices of dying individuals and their close companions.

In its earliest forms in the UK, the hospice movement, developed by Cicely Saunders, was a visionary and innovative response to the neglect of pain relief observed among dying cancer patients (Clark 1998; Clark and Seymour 1999). Developments in the US took a different form, reflecting the greater cultural preoccupation with individualism in that country (Field 1996). Kübler-Ross's description of 'Death: The final stage of growth' (1975) perhaps best captures the voice of the hospice movement as it developed in the US, in which psychological preparation for death was enhanced by a 'sharing of knowledge' (1975: 32) with dying people and their companions. The 'right to be heard' (1975: 7) was promoted by Kübler-Ross as the cornerstone of the reclaiming of death from an event that is lonely, impersonal and medicalized, to one surrounded by 'rest, peace and dignity' (1975: 8).

Seale (1995a,b) suggests that the various narratives surrounding dying may be appropriated actively and reflexively by individuals to ascribe meaning to their own and others' dying. However, as Seale (1995a,b) observes, the maintenance of these predominant narratives depends critically on conditions of 'self-awareness' and 'knowledge' of the certainty of dying: conditions that do not appertain for many deaths which occur within late modern society. While Seale draws attention to deaths occurring in extreme old age where dementia, confusion and institutionalization frequently herald dying, deaths occurring under the auspices of high technology in the intensive care unit are possibly the examples *par excellence* of the 'unnatural' medicalized event which all the 'good' death narratives logically exclude.

Conclusion

In this chapter I have attempted to set the scene for the empirical chapters that follow by introducing the various bodies of literature that informed the study design and influenced the formulation of its research questions. Each of these bodies of literature are drawn on further in subsequent discussions. The research questions underpinning the study were as follows:

1 What are the social interactions involved in the process whereby a decision is made to withdraw life-supporting care in intensive care?
2 What are the concepts of a 'good death' held by different groups in the intensive care environment, and where do these ideas originate?

3 How do healthcare staff assess and respond to the needs of patients' significant others and how is this care perceived by the recipients?
4 How do healthcare staff make sense of their close proximity to dying and death? Do they employ particular 'coping' strategies?

These questions acted as a guide to the conduct of the study, aiding the direction of attention during observation and interviewing but with the overarching aim of achieving a multi-layered analysis of the way in which death and dying are interpreted and managed within one highly specialized area of the modern hospital. Intensive care is a microcosm of the rapidly changing cultural, legal, ethical and clinical environment that attends death in modern society. While it may be considered as a cultural expression of medical rationality, it is an area that has frequently to confront and contain the human suffering and sadness associated with death. The way in which the tensions between 'science' and 'compassion' are resolved is the focus of the chapters that follow.

Notes

1 Intermittent positive pressure ventilation refers to the mechanical ventilation of the lungs via a tracheostomy or an endo-tracheal tube.
2 The 'iron lung' is a colloquial term used to describe the 'cuirass ventilator' in which negative pressure applied to the thorax is used to produce artificial ventilation.
3 Examples of technological innovations that have become part of 'ordinary' practice are the use of syringe drivers, cardiac monitoring and pulse oximetry.
4 Multiple organ failure is diagnosed when three or more organs require intensive therapy: either pharmacologically or mechanically. The combination of heart, respiratory and renal failure would be an example.

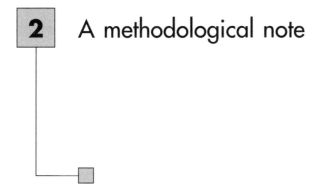

2 | A methodological note

The original idea for conducting a piece of ethnographic research of this nature was the result of years of experience of nursing work in intensive care units together with some personal experience of acute illness in my immediate family. I wanted, although this was not formulated clearly in my mind at the outset, to enhance my own understanding of events that I had found troubling and disturbing. Completing and 'writing up' the study has, perhaps, also been a way of drawing a metaphorical line under my previous life as an intensive care nurse.

My first awareness of intensive care and its powerful combination of risk and hope came when my father was admitted to intensive care following heart surgery in 1976. I was unable to visit him there since his operation coincided with my first few days as an undergraduate at University, but I can remember clearly the anxiety of waiting for news, and the relief when I was told that he had been transferred safely to an ordinary ward. Following completion of a social science degree, I decided to train as a nurse and found myself working at a large London teaching hospital. Several years later, a combination of choice and circumstantial opportunity found me completing specialist nurse training in general intensive care and working eventually as a sister in a small intensive therapy unit in a district general hospital just outside London. Following a break to look after my children, I returned to work in another intensive therapy unit, where I worked for four years (1990–1994). I came back to nursing work at this time with, possibly, a more critical 'eye' since I had studied for a part-time Master's degree in sociology during my childcare break. In some ways I felt that I was rather an outsider: a nurse but also a sociologist, looking in on myself acting a role within a very strange environment. Further, the intersection of the personal and professional had been very forcibly imprinted on my mind during 1989, when my 3-year-old son became gravely ill with epiglottitis, resulting in an obstructed airway. He was treated quickly and expertly in a paediatric intensive care unit, but it took a long time to recover from the near brush with death. Subsequently I felt better able to empathize with the experiences of those with whom I came into contact during my professional work, and developed a particular interest in how the care of and management of dying patients was perceived by their companions and families.

Looking back on my working life in intensive care, the incidents, events and people that I remember most clearly tend to be associated with death. It was on this experiential level that I was aware of what appeared to be inevitable problems regarding the uncertainty of prognosis. In particular there seemed to be intransigent difficulties caused by the apparently very different perspectives of nursing and medicine regarding not only the recognition of dying, but also the most appropriate ways to manage the care and treatment of those patients who were probably dying. These problems, by the time I left intensive care, seemed set to become more entrenched and complicated. It was at a time when the availability increased of highly invasive treatments for multiple organ failure and yet when financial, legal and ethical pressures were reaching previously unknown proportions. This autobiographical 'baggage' (Harvey 1994: 137) was to play a critical part both in the conduct of the study and in my interpretation of the case-study data. It also fashioned the conceptual slant of my work towards highlighting issues of broad theoretical interest while at the same time representing the 'real' and immediate consequences of those issues for individuals involved with dying people in intensive care.

Research design: using the case study as an ethical framework

The methodological literature pointed to the use of the case-study design (Yin 1984) as a means of examining the 'micro-mediation' (Platt 1983: 11) of social processes within intensive care while simultaneously enabling, as Platt puts it, 'the reader to grasp the meaning of the data presented and the lives they stand for . . . (and) also [to] give holistic accounts of events or life-patterns which show social supports or constraints' (1983: 6). An argument put forward by Mitchell that highlighted the analytical value of 'accumulated experience and knowledge' (Mitchell 1983: 203) of a social setting in drawing wider inferences from case-study research was particularly persuasive given my familiarity with the setting.

While these methodological factors underpinned the research design, equally important influences were the practical and ethical issues that had to be addressed. Access was relatively straightforward given my previous professional role in the area and the fact that one of the chosen fieldwork sites was a former work area, although this in itself gave rise to methodological problems that had to be faced later on. Permission to access both units was arranged following an appointment to see the medical director and clinical nurse manager, at which time the proposal and research ethics committee submission was presented and discussed. Letters were sent to the nursing, medical and paramedical staff giving them a brief outline of the study and inviting them to discuss any concerns they had at one of several meetings arranged before the fieldwork started. During these meetings the way in which I would act as an observer was worked out and the details of a consent process were clarified.

Looking first at the consent process, it was decided to gain consent for observation from the healthcare staff responsible for the patients and from those individuals designated as the patient's 'next of kin', whether this was a family member or a close companion. Consent for follow-up interviews after the discharge or death of the patient from intensive care was to be gained separately by means of a letter sent to those individuals who had agreed to further contact.

In some respects attempting to get a form of 'proxy' consent for observation was an unusual path to follow: consent by proxy for adults has no legal status (Dimond 1990), and might be criticized as merely an attempt to conform to standard practice and ease the conscience of the uneasy researcher. While I cannot deny that such concerns *were* present, special circumstances also made it imperative that clearly laid down, and highly visible 'rules' were formulated. At the time that the research was being planned, sensitivity about the extreme vulnerability of intensive care patients, which was already heightened as a result of the case of Beverley Allitt, reached new levels of anxiety. A well-publicized case was just coming to awareness (Foster 1994), which involved the alleged interference with life-support equipment by an intensive care staff nurse at a hospital in Northern England. The nurses at both of the intensive care units involved in this study were thoroughly shaken by the news and this remained a topic of conversation during the whole of the fieldwork period.

Further, I hoped that building a consent process into the observational phase of the fieldwork would foster sustained 'engagement' – in keeping with the ethnographic tradition – between myself, the patient's healthcare staff and family and friends. I knew that to have any chance of achieving a 'credible' account of an environment about which I already had my own preconceptions I had to try to enter the experience of others and do so as closely and intensively as possible. Asking to share in people's experiences in a very 'up front' way, seemed the best approach to doing this quickly and efficiently. I was to come to realize that it was the consent procedure that had the most influence on the way in which I was 'seen' by the research participants. It was critical in determining the degree of rapport that developed between us, and it influenced crucially the character of the roles I was to adopt in the wider fieldwork setting.

Turning to my observational role, there were obvious problems of conducting research in an area where I had developed a great deal of 'taken for granted' knowledge. Developing a research role would give rise to problems of role identity and, potentially, a clash of nurse and researcher responsibilities (Field 1991; Punch 1994; Holloway and Wheeler 1995). In an attempt to create a space between nurse and researcher it was agreed therefore that I would not undertake hands on care; and that I would not observe the delivery of intimate physical care. My role was to be that of a general helper: answering telephones, taking messages, clearing trolleys, fetching and carrying. It was also hoped that this plan would further preserve the privacy of each patient and prevent my identification by their companions as a nurse with responsibility for the care of their relative. In spite of these plans at times I found myself being asked, or expected, to behave as a nurse. It quickly became clear that if I was to retain the trust and respect of my former colleagues then I had to be seen to help with their work. The manner in which this help was given became crucial in order to retain my researcher role while at the same time preserving the bond between the healthcare staff and myself. Any other path would, I felt, have been false and insincere. Such familiarity brought other methodological problems: for example, I was not always able to 'pull off' asking questions about events in the way that a 'naive' observer may have been able to do. Such questioning aroused incredulity that I should have 'forgotten' in such a short space of time that which was taken for granted. I either had to choose carefully those to whom I addressed questions or sometimes act as the scatter-brained academic to get anywhere with such enquiries.

My experiences and thoughts during the fieldwork can be illustrated by one example, drawn from the case-study data, which focuses in particular on the relationship I developed with the wife and son of a dying man. This was the first case study I completed, and perhaps as a result I came to regard it as somehow special. I built up a particularly close relationship with the two main figures in the case study: something that in no way was a common feature of all the cases.

'Jack Hart' was a 74-year-old man who was admitted to intensive care following a severe head injury sustained during a road traffic accident. His next of kin were his wife 'Mary' and his son 'Michael'. I gained consent from Mary and Michael to follow Jack's illness on day two of his intensive care admission, completing seven days of observation and conducting four follow-up interviews.

I identified Jack as a possible inclusion in the study a few hours after his admission to intensive care.[1] I agreed with Helen, Jack's primary nurse that I could keep in contact with her over the next 24 hours and that during this time she would assess whether she thought that his wife and son could withstand the extra 'burden' of being asked to share their experiences with me. We agreed that she would check that they had been interviewed by the senior medical staff and had time to make some sense of the information given to them before I made any contact.

Helen introduced me to Mary and Michael at 11 am the next day, 35 hours after Jack's admission to intensive care. Helen at this point has already checked with them that they do not mind being introduced to a 'researcher from the University' who would like to ask their permission to observe the planning and delivery of care to Jack, as well as talking to them about their experiences if they feel able. This latter point is seized upon by Mary, who Helen reports to me later says, 'Yes, yes, anything to take my mind off what is happening' and 'I need someone to talk to – perhaps she will talk to me'.

So it is that, albeit unbeknown to me, the pattern of my relationship with Mary, and through her with Michael, is formed by Mary's early interpretation of what I might be able to do to help her. I become quickly and forcibly aware of Mary's hopes. She grasps my hand as I am introduced to her and her son, and continues to sit holding my hand while pouring out everything that has happened since she first received the news of Jack's accident. Both she and Michael cry at various points during her account. Eventually, however, both Mary and Michael smile as they recount to me the kinds of interests Jack had, and the kinds of things they had done as a family together. It is sometime later that Michael turns to me – almost as an aside – and asks if I want to explain about the research I am doing, and it is only at this point that I am able to begin to explain my research intentions to them. Michael reads the information sheet about the study very carefully and asks several questions. Mary on the other hand, seems already to have decided that I can 'do what you like dear', and it feels like a struggle to get her to listen to what I am saying while I go through the information sheet verbally with her. The problems of gaining 'informed consent' in such a situation are thrown into sharp focus: Mary, it seemed, had developed her own particular view of who I was and what I was going to do. The formality of the information sheet impinged little on her view of me and on her understanding of the research. Thus that the relational aspect of the research was highlighted, and I began to develop some formative understanding of the complex issues I would meet during the coming months.

Later the same day, while I am sitting writing field notes in the staff rest room, Jack's nurse comes in to ask if I could help her by sitting with Mary. She explains that she is busy with Jack, and can ill afford any time away from his bed. I wrote the following at this time:

*After the **lunchtime handover** from the early to the late staff I decide to leave for a while. I get the feeling that Y the student nurse is feeling stressed by my presence. As I am writing notes in the coffee room the door opens and Y comes in: 'I hope you don't mind, but Mrs Hart is asking if someone could sit with her . . .' I quickly say that of course I* *don't mind, but **am** wondering how this stands vis à vis my research. As I walk out of the room towards the waiting room I decide that, having made contact earlier on, I am morally bound to answer Mrs Hart's need.*

(From the field notes – day 1)

My relationship with Mary and Michael over the following days develops such that I feel that I am perceived by them as an interested friend, and perhaps potential nurse: someone to whom they voice thoughts or possibly merely pass the time of day during the hours and hours of waiting and sitting they have to endure. On day four for example, Michael talks to me at some length while his mother is having a rest. He gives me some insight into the tangle of worries and fears about the present and the future that he is having to face:

*At 7 pm I sit and have a conversation with Michael, Mary has gone for a sleep. He tells me quite a lot about his work; but then suddenly changes the subject: 'I don't **want him** to survive and be like that chap from the Hillsborough disaster – she [Mary] won't grieve properly **until** he dies . . . and I need to know what comes next and no one seems to be able to tell us. Will we have to get a bed ready at home or will he stay here? . . . seems a funny thing to say about your Dad, but I did get on with him, I liked **him**. He could be gruff, but he entertained me – he was a friend.'*

(From the field notes – day 4)

Some days later, after Jack's transfer from intensive care to the general ward, I make regular visits to see Michael and Mary. Jack by this time is clearly dying, and all his various supportive treatments have been withdrawn. It becomes increasingly difficult to retain any sense of 'doing research' at this time, and although I continue to write field notes, I feel my focus has shifted to a more straightforward matter of person-to-person concern and compassion:

*11.30 am I go to the ward to see if I am allowed to see Michael and Mary. The staff nurse directs me to go to room 8. It's a long ward and room 8 is at the bottom and round the corner. The blind is down on the door and I hesitate for a minute before tilting slightly the metal handle that controls the blind, I can see Michael and Mary in the room . . . Michael comes and opens the door. They are pleased to see **me** but I notice immediately how pale and tired they are. Mary is tearful: 'I'm a **bit** upset today Jane, I keep trying not to cry . . . but look at **him**, he looked so lovely and peaceful up there, and now look – he doesn't look like **my little** man any more . . . we're on our own now, no one popping past and stopping for a chat'*

(From the field notes – day 9)

Jack dies two days later, shortly after his wife and son have left the ward briefly for a rest.

Several months later both Mary and Michael agree to me visiting them at home to conduct an interview about their experiences. Retrospective interviewing in this way provided another opportunity to incorporate individual accounts of 'lived experience' into the case-study data. It also provided an alternative perspective on the observational data, and allowed some conclusions to be drawn about the impact of the intensive care experience on the ability to make sense of death and serious illness. Michael's account of events shortly after his father's transfer to the ward fills in a 'gap' in the story that would not have been possible otherwise:

> *Michael*: er, when we got down to the ward and we first saw him – I think it were in the morning he had been transferred I think and he hadn't had his wash and such, and he looked horrible he looked awful. It upset me mother a lot, er, there were a staff nurse sat on there and she said, 'don't be upset too much', she says, 'go and have a cup of tea or something, go and have your dinner', she said because he would be having like his normal afternoon wash and when you see him again his hair will be combed and everything. [She said] It's just because of the transfer . . . because its a surgical ward we haven't got time or the care that they've got up there, but next time don't worry, when you see him soon he will be all right. And when we did come back he was as right as rain, which took a lot of pressure off
>
> (From retrospective interview)

At times the interview data gave further methodological insight into the way in which I had been regarded during the observational period. Michael and Mary, in separate responses to a naively worded question about what had been helpful on intensive care tell me:

> *Michael*: well, I hope it don't make you big-headed, but you were . . . I mean, I know it's a study you were doing and all, but you asking questions and getting answers definitely helped . . . to have that extra were definitely a help
>
> *Mary*: you were very helpful, just being you, just being there with me . . . I talked to you a lot about his life and all we did and got up to, told you all about my life as well
>
> (From retrospective interview)

The extent to which such responses were a product of the unusual social situation of the interview, or an attempt to make me feel comfortable is, of course, open to question. Similarly a number of other issues and concerns are raised by such recollections: issues that I have never fully resolved in my mind. Hence, this chapter concludes with some questions and thoughts that seem to flow from both this particular case and from the research more generally, all of which I think have wider relevance to ethnographic research at the end of life:

How is the role of 'researcher' to be fashioned in the face of the human experience of death and dying?

My experience of doing this piece of work has highlighted how important it is to have a debate about these issues. Clearly, such work can be illuminating and can aid the production of knowledge in a field where we understand relatively little about the mechanics of delivering end-of-life care and making critical decisions about life and death. However, no one should underestimate the grave responsibility they incur when undertaking such work. Unlike the more focused modes of clinical research where attention is directed at a discrete issue, and the boundaries of activity are clear, ethnographic research can be as messy and tangled as everyday life. Issues associated with risk, trust and expectation arise constantly, many of which may not have been previously thought about and to which a response is required 'on the hoof'. The risks of getting it wrong are considerable, and it is highly likely that we will never know whether what was done was appropriate and reasonable. Ethnographic research is essentially an exercise in social relationships: in the field of death and dying such relationships can be both fraught and fragile. In this context, the process of doing such work becomes just as important as the purposes and aims that have given rise to the study, and the outcomes it is hoped that will follow.

Where is the voice of the patient in this type of work?

In many ways, the experience of intensive care from the patient's perspective does not feature in this book. This absence of patients' voices has been noted as a problem in studies of this kind, most notably by those who have had experience themselves of critical illness and have written about it later (Rier 2000). The most usual way of accessing patients' perspectives is to interview them retrospectively (see, for example, Hall-Smith et al. 1997). My study design, and the purposive sampling of people who were most likely to die, threw considerable obstacles in the path of this particular route of investigation. However, I have tried to represent the day-to-day contact of the intensive care staff with critically ill people in a manner that renders their personhood highly visible. However, I acknowledge a 'gap' in my account and echo calls for a debate about how this might be bridged in a manner that is ethically sound.

How is 'informed consent' pursued with the companions of dying people in prospective studies of this kind?

I am not convinced on the basis of my experiences that this is possible in this type of work. However, I do think that recent commentaries on 'process consent' (see, for example, Usher and Arthur 1998) are useful, insofar as they point out that what is important and possible is a renewing of the contract between researcher and researched at regular intervals. I also think that it is possible to be as candid as possible with people about what you are trying to achieve, and, even if this is only fairly approximate, what you will be asking of them. However, it is certainly true that 'once and for all' consent cannot be taken as read, even when the safe practices of filling out a consent sheet have been followed.

Is there any role for 'proxy consent' in this type of study?

I think in my particular study there was a good case, even though my attention in many ways was not so much focused on the patient, but on those surrounding him or her. It acted as a form of reminder that I no longer had a right of access by dint of my professional role and was a safeguard against covertness in a situation where it was essential that everyone knew and understood what I was doing. However, I do think that the consent process as a whole sometimes raised issues with patients' families that they were probably trying not to think about. To this extent, it was unfair on those who coped by trying to distance themselves from the harsh realities of their situation. I think, however, that most of these people either said 'no' at an early stage, or my access to them was the subject of 'gatekeeping' by the nursing staff.

What might be the costs of participation in research of this kind?

Clearly there are costs to the participants that have to be balanced with the wider purposes of the research: issues of distress, unfulfilled expectations, unwitting breaches of confidentiality and anonymity; these are some of the risks for those who take part in such studies. However, there are also costs for the researcher: I can remember feeling a bit like a parasite when doing this study, and, although I don't think I recognized it at the time, suffered from a moderate degree of stress. I was lucky to have good support: I'm not sure that everyone gets what is needed in this regard.

To what extent is it possible to preserve anonymity given the detail of this data – is the researcher solely responsible for such preservation?

In my PhD *viva*, one of the examiners pointed this issue out, saying that some fairly unsophisticated detective work on the part of someone reading my thesis could enable them to identify relatively easily both where the research was conducted and who was involved. I think this is probably true, and leads to two conclusions: first, when and how such work is reported and written up for publication is critical; and second, we as a research community must agree not to attempt, or to encourage, detective work of this kind. In this case some years have elapsed since the observations were recorded, and I have tried as far as possible to conceal identities and places.

Note

1 The critically ill individuals at the centre of each case study were selected purposively so that those at highest risk of death were followed. Individuals fell into two groups: first, those who had an APACHE II severity of illness score of 24 points or above (Knaus *et al*. 1985), giving a statistical risk of death of 73 per cent; and second, those who (according to a clinical assessment on admission) were predicted to be unlikely to survive. Only individuals who had been admitted between 24 and 72 hours previously would be followed. Several exclusion criteria were stated:

1 All those who had been in Intensive Care for less than 24 hours.
2 All those who were under the age of 18.
3 All those who were thought to be 'brain dead'.
4 All those without a designated next of kin.

3 | Medical knowledge in intensive care: constructing prognostic certainty

Patients are admitted into intensive care from several sources. They may come from the Accident and Emergency department following an acute episode of illness or collapse at home; they may be transferred as an emergency from a general ward (possibly from another hospital) following an acute deterioration in their condition, or they may arrive straight from the operating theatre following major surgery or an unexpected complication during more routine surgery. In the early days following a patient's admission to intensive care, medical staff are faced with the task of achieving a measure of diagnostic and prognostic certainty with which to formulate future treatment (or non-treatment) plans. This process can take many hours and days, and is complicated by the fact that almost all patients admitted to intensive care are unable, by virtue of the severity of their illness and the nature of the treatments administered to them, to communicate verbally with their clinicians.

This chapter follows Atkinson (1995), and charts the way in which medical staff assemble and 'read' clinical data from a complex range of sources, highlighting the role of medical specialization in this process. It explores how a shared meaning of that data is negotiated in terms that define patients as either 'dying' or 'recoverable', and how a framework is developed to guide and delimit future medical action.

The first part of the chapter examines the way in which accounts are established of 'health history' and 'quality of life'[1] when a patient is first admitted to intensive care. These concepts are revealed as key parameters influencing the interpretation of clinical data and the direction of medical action in intensive care.

The second part of the chapter explores the 'routine' use of the ward round and medical notes both as a means of legitimating 'technological' knowledge about the bodies of ill people and as a framework for organizing clinical work in intensive care. The discussion here has been influenced by a concept of 'the body' as a product of certain types of knowledge (Armstrong 1983a; Anspach 1987; May 1992a,b; Slomka 1992; Lupton 1994), in which the physiological reality of certain conditions is given social meaning within particular healthcare settings (Wright and Treacher 1982; Muller and Koenig 1988).

Establishing accounts of health history and quality of life

The attempt to compile a health history of each individual is an ongoing feature of clinical work in intensive care, but features particularly strongly in the preliminary assessment that is completed soon after admission. Obtaining this information is crucial since it helps to determine the character and extent of the intensive therapies that are commenced in each person's case, having far-reaching effects on the eventual 'cascade' (Slomka 1992: 252) of decisions that are taken concerning the withdrawal or continuation of that treatment. Running alongside attempts to formulate a comprehensive picture of health history is work to unravel the nature of the patients' presenting condition. In many cases this will be a complex combination of acute and chronic pathology, which, in order to be untangled, requires both the opinion of various medical specialists and the extensive application of diagnostic technology. A key concept employed during this diagnostic 'detective' work is that of 'quality of life', interpreted by intensive care staff as the potential ability of the individual to return to meaningful social functioning.

In an observational study of junior medical staff within general hospital environments in the US, Muller and Koenig (1988) highlight the problem of assessing the potential capacity of unconscious individuals to return to a 'normal' level of social functioning. They suggest that in such a situation, medical staff have recourse to two other sources of data, expert knowledge about disease and familiarity with the ill person:

> In those situations where patients are mentally impaired and unable to communicate with their care-takers; physicians, on the basis of their knowledge of disease processes and outcomes, as well as their familiarity with individual patients, evaluate patients' potential for resuming social roles or interacting in a meaningful way with others in their environment.
>
> (Muller and Koenig 1988: 359)

Such information is not, however, always readily available about those individuals admitted to intensive care. There is usually no previous familiarity between the patient and the intensive care staff, and in the case of accident and emergency admissions, no familiarity between the patient and other medical specialists involved in their treatment. Further, the presenting condition of some patients may be of a complexity that confounds the most expert attempts to unravel its nature and likely outcome. Some individuals may be briefly conscious on arrival in the intensive care units but in such an extreme state of ill health that rapid sedation and ventilation is necessitated. This precludes the exchange of any information with the healthcare staff about their previous state of health, about their opinion regarding their quality of life or preferences for care and treatment. The influence of this on medical practice and on the problems of defining 'dying' can be illustrated by the words of one consultant anaesthetist who discussed with me the problems of 'knowing' what an individual's 'normal' condition is:

> 'It's notoriously difficult – of course sometimes it's easy for me, as consultant, to look at a patient and say: "Why have they come in here, they're not an ITU patient, they got this wrong and that wrong" – but for the registrar and the senior registrar faced with a patient in casualty, that information is not always available. The problem becomes one of treatment. My opinion is that once you know someone is chronically ill then you give them maximal treatment, like anyone else, for a period of time, perhaps 24–36 hours, and then you take a clear decision to withdraw. I'm not into this half-hearted, well we'll do this but not that – that can prolong things for a long, long time. I prefer a clear decision to be made. Some of my colleagues do not agree with me and that's when it becomes difficult.' [Intensive care consultant]

(From field notes)

In some cases, there may be some familiarity between the ill person and members of the wider medical team responsible for their care prior to admission to intensive care. However, as we shall see, this background knowledge may be interpreted by the intensive care medical staff as partial, or even 'misleading'.

Material from three of the case studies will be used to illustrate these points. The first case demonstrates the difficulties of interpreting clinical data collected shortly after the ill person's admission, showing how this interpretation is dependent on achieving what is, for the intensive care medical staff, a 'reliable' view of that person's previous health history. The second case focuses on achieving an agreed definition of 'quality of life' in the face of several possible interpretations of the concept. The third case demonstrates the critical impact of the interpretation of health history and quality of life on the delimitation, or narrowing, of medical action. It illustrates the way in which aspects of the individual's condition are isolated into long-term, 'chronic' features, the management of which is then placed *outside* the delineated area of responsibility of intensive care.

Case study 1 Achieving an account of health history

Mrs Hall was a 79-year-old woman who was admitted to hospital with an acute confusional state and respiratory failure. She had become progressively ill over a three-week period inspite of receiving treatment from her general practitioner. Her adult children had alerted the GP following a rapid deterioration in her condition and she was brought by ambulance to the Accident and Emergency department. She was formally admitted under the care of a team of physicians but was quickly admitted to intensive care following an urgent referral from the Accident and Emergency staff to the duty anaesthetist for assistance.

The duty anaesthetist described her involvement with Mrs Hall in the Accident and Emergency Department ('Cas') during a conversation with me two days later:

'*I got called to Cas. on Wednesday to tube her and had to take over – I really didn't get the chance to work out all the pathology and the physiology but I did a few things which worked and she improved slightly – I 'phoned the SR [senior registrar] for advice – he laughed when I said she was 79 – but said that it was up to me to make the decision about what it was best to do. He said that was the way to learn. So I said, right, well, I want to bring her up to the unit, ventilate her for 24 hours and see how she goes. He agreed and that's what we did.*'

(From field notes)

Here we can see how the junior doctor has to embark on life-preserving interventions with an almost complete absence of information about the broader context of Mrs Hall's condition, and also in the situation of an apparent lack of any policy regarding the admission of older people to intensive care.[2] Once Mrs Hall is admitted to the intensive care unit, the problem of unravelling her health history becomes urgent: a mass of clinical data is now becoming available about her. So at this point the notes function as an important means of summarizing the information available, pointing to 'gaps' or inconsistencies in knowledge, and allowing medical staff to communicate with each other. Moreover, the group activity of 'reading the notes' during the ward rounds can be seen as a means of negotiating the meaning of the data presented within them, and as a means of defining the most appropriate course of future medical action.

The following is an extract from the notes written about Mrs Hall on her admission to intensive care:

(1) '*Fit and well*' until 3 weeks ago, not seen a doctor in 20 years.
(2) '*Flu-like*' symptoms. Saw GP, diuretic given for swollen ankles and slight shortness of breath. Since then, deterioration and confusion.

(3) *Previous smoker. No known previous illness. On admission,*
     moribund:
(4)   *– rr 30+ in respiratory failure*
(5)   *– unresponsive, GCS 5–7*
(6)   *– cool peripheries*
(7)   *– bounding pulse – 140 irregular; bp 125/70*
(8)   *– dehydrated*
(9)   *– chest creps*
(10)   *– elective intubation – transfer itu*
(11)   *– pulsatile liver, JVP up, tricuspid regurgitation*
(12) *On itu admission chest x-ray shows old changes r. upper lobe?*
(13)   *fibrotic lung disease*
(14) *Renal impairment (? new, ? longstanding)*
(15) *Required DC synchronised shock 50j for tachycardia 150.*
(16) *Blood results – K 6.7*
(17)   *Urea   – 25.5*
(18)   *Creat – 163*
(19)   *PH   – 6.9*
(20) PCO_2 *– 14.24*
(21) PO_2 *– 33.52*
(22) HCO_3 *– 16.9*
(23)   *BE   – 9.7*
(24) *? Chest infection on top of dilated cardiomyopathy.*

13/7/95 Senior Registrar review (chest medicine)
Very ill lady – probable septic shock with elements of hypovalaemia at
presentation: multiple organ failure makes things difficult and adds
adverse factors towards prognosis. Recommend – amiodarone/dopamine
Gentamicin for i/v cover. Staining for AFB (old tb from cxr)

(Intensive care staff entry)
IPPV 40 per cent, dopamine and dobutamine (C.O. 4.1, SVR 1805)
Cefuroxime, gentamicin, clindomycin.
TPN and ng feeding (referred dietician.)
Referred to cardiologists re. amiodarone – they recommend miodarone
and digoxin.

(From the medical notes)

Here we have an account of Mrs Hall that combines a number of features. The most outstanding of these is the brevity of the notes – her past history, her current state and the plans for her treatment are outlined in a succinct way, using medical shorthand: for example, 'rr' denotes respiratory rate, 'GCS' means 'Glasgow Coma Scale', and JVP refers to jugular venous pressure. Mrs Hall is, apparently, reinterpreted as a list of medical/technical problems, which can be enumerated and measured. We can also see that information gathered from Mrs Hall's family or from her GP has been marked by inverted commas (lines 1 and 2), giving a sense to the reader that this is not information to be relied on. What follows subsequently is not, however, marked in this way and is presented uncritically as fact. This characteristic 'marking' of information that is seen as potentially unreliable has been observed by Anspach (1988), in an analysis of the language used during case presentations, and also by Atkinson (1995), in a study of haematology specialists.

The data summarized in the notes can be partitioned into that obtained by clinical, hands-on examination, and that obtained by clinical investigation. For example, in lines numbered 4–11 the information presented comes entirely from the bedside examination of Mrs Hall. This is followed by an interpretation of a chest X-ray film (line 12) where the question mark used illustrates the problematic nature of 'reading' such investigations in the absence of comprehensive information about the individual's previous health. The problem of interpretation comes into play again over the question of renal impairment (line 14): is this impairment a new feature of her condition or a long-standing problem? Lower down, (line 24) the possible diagnosis of a chest infection with dilated cardiomyopathy is mooted and the advice of the specialist in chest medicine is apparently sought. His entry confirms the severity of Mrs Hall's condition and gives some guidance as to the management of her drugs and the direction of future investigations. He raises the possibility here of reactivated tubercular disease based on his interpretation of Mrs Hall's chest X-ray. This early collaboration with another team of doctors illustrates the specialized nature of medical work – opinions and information are gathered and compiled by various individuals and teams of individuals many of whom may have only a fleeting contact with the ill person, or only have access to their tissue samples, or body images (Atkinson 1995).

On the first day of observation in Mrs Hall's case, a ward round takes place in the afternoon during which some time is spent discussing her health history and reading the entries in the notes. Some of the characteristic features observed in the the clinical notes re-occur in this exclusively verbal exchange between four doctors, and again it is possible to see the impact of formative judgements about Mrs Hall's *past* health problems on the *present* interpretation of clinical data that have become available:

Consultant 1 and the registrar talk together and discuss blood results and the possibility of legionella infection and what her previous state of health was.

Consultant 1: 'It's so difficult to tell, we've spoken to two separate members of her family and they both deny that she has been ill at all – and yet I think she must have been. Her X-ray is so abnormal, and apparently she hasn't been going outside'.

The senior registrar and Consultant 2 stand a few feet away from the others, and have their backs to them. They are discussing the cardiovascular data and are trying to manipulate the monitor to gather more data.

(From the field notes)

Again the problem of aligning the information given by family members with that obtained by clinical investigations occurs. Mrs Hall's family 'deny' that she has been ill but this denial is treated as suspect because of, first, the abnormal appearance of the chest X-ray and, second, the report from the family that she has not been going outside. Presumably the family do not regard this as a sign of illness, but to the medical staff it becomes a significant sign that points to underlying pathology. This treatment of 'lay' information and definitions of illness as suspect allows the medical staff to draw the boundaries around what is reliable knowledge: i.e. that gained through their direct examination or investigation. The nursing staff (who have not, up until now, contributed to the discussion) suggest that Mrs Hall may have abdominal pain. The basis on which they deduce this is from their observations of her level of comfort during the care that they give to her. These observations are more akin to an intuitive sense, rather than being the more formal approach of medical, physical examination, but are taken seriously by the medical staff because they have already established that she has an enlarged liver and possible hepatitis. It is proposed that an ultrasound of Mrs Hall's abdomen should be ordered. This illustrates the way in which a wide range of signs is reported by different parties but is taken up in varying ways by the medical staff according to their own theories.

The end result of the ward round is a brief entry in the notes in which the current knowledge about Mrs Hall is summarized and a plan of action outlined thus:

Improving cardiac function
Acute – on chronic respiratory failure – weaning problem.
Liver congestion +/– hepatitis ?cause
G.I. bleed.
Add ranitidine/ frusemide/ micro-review.
Continue respiratory support. Ultrasound abdomen and gastroscopy. Albumin, diuretics, phosphates. Noradrenaline for low svr. Reduce dobutamine.

(From the medical notes)

In Mrs Hall's case, her previous contact with the medical world had been limited, the contributions from her family apparently vague and the information from the general practitioner scanty. It is left up to the intensive care staff to assemble their version of her health history which best fits with their own perspective on events. In other cases, where there has been more extensive contact with medicine, this process of assembly is more complicated.

The next case focuses on the management of a woman who was transferred from a general medical ward into intensive care on the basis of an assessment by the referring physician that her previous quality of life was good. The subsequent difference in opinion over the accuracy of this assessment is illustrated, showing how critical is the impact of such an evaluation in directing the formulation of treatment plans in those cases where recovery is acknowledged as unlikely.

Case study 2 Assessing quality of life

Mrs Richards was a 73-year-old woman who, prior to her admission to intensive care, had been on an orthopaedic ward in Eastern hospital for one week undergoing investigations for her severe back pain. She had fallen at home two years previously resulting in fractures to her femur, wrist and hand and the orthopaedic team was concerned that her back pain was related to this accident. Mrs Richards's condition gradually deteriorated on the orthopaedic ward and a diagnosis of pneumonia and septicaemia was made. She was admitted to intensive care for ventilation and circulatory support after suffering an acute deterioration in her cardio-respiratory condition. The admission was negotiated by a consultant physician to whom Mrs Richards had been referred by the orthopaedic team. Shortly after her admission to the intensive care unit, and during the process of nursing assessment, her primary nurse was told by Mrs Richards's daughter, Susan, that she had been largely dependent on a wheelchair since suffering a stroke and needed help with day-to-day tasks and meals. Susan felt that she was suffering from depression and had 'no purpose in life' since the death of her husband for whom she had cared during 15 years of 'horrendous ill-health.' (Susan's words as reported by the primary nurse.)

Forty hours after Mrs Richards's admission, the team of physicians who had made the earlier referral, visits her on the unit. The consultant physician seems surprised and angry to hear the report from the intensive care staff about her poor quality of life at home. He rounds on his registrar, who was responsible for the transfer arrangements made for Mrs Richards:

'I thought you said she was fit?'[3] (Turning to his registrar.) His registrar looks uncomfortable. Quickly, they (the physicians and anaesthetists) start to discuss the source of her sepsis – she has a staphylococcal infection in her blood which has affected her circulation and she is needing multiple drugs to keep up her blood pressure – dopamine, dobutamine, noradrenaline and vasopressin.

(From the field notes)

This extract illustrates the problems faced by medical staff in attempting to make urgent clinical decisions in the context of information that they see as inaccurate about an individual's chances of responding to treatment. The physician's anger at discovering that Mrs Richards has been, in his view, perhaps admitted inappropriately may be partly due to his desire to appear trustworthy to his intensive care colleagues. The reality of this fear is substantiated by the attitude of the intensive care consultant who says later to his intensive care colleagues: *'I think we were seriously misled about how fit this lady was'*. The implication of this statement is that perhaps they would not have agreed to her admission had a more accurate picture of her life at home been available to them. Given that she is now under their care and that very substantial treatments have already been instigated – namely maximal drug therapy and 100 per cent oxygen – they must decide on further management while continuing to search for a cause of her sepsis. A 'middle course' is charted, which takes into account the complex moral and practical differences between withholding treatment (i.e. not starting in the first place) and withdrawing treatment already commenced.[4] It is agreed that renal support would: *'probably not be given'* and *'perhaps we ought not to try too hard'* (senior registrar: reported in the field notes).

The next case illustrates the way in which therapeutic options are narrowed on the basis of an understanding of 'health history' and 'quality of life'. We see how possible avenues of treatment are considered and subjected to an interrogation that focuses on the possibility of their long-term success rather than their short-term efficacy. In this way, disease processes are subdivided into 'irrecoverable' and 'recoverable', and a basis for difficult non-treatment decisions legitimitated.

Case study 3 Narrowing therapeutic options

Mr Albert Randall, a 62-year-old man, was admitted to the intensive care unit at Western hospital for cardiac and ventilatory support following surgery for a perforated duodenal ulcer. Four days before his transfer to intensive care, Mr Randall had been admitted to a medical ward after a referral from his general practitioner. Mr Randall's wife, Enid, had called the general practitioner when she realized that Mr Randall was vomiting blood. During his stay on the medical ward, Mr Randall received an exploratory gastroscopy, a blood transfusion, and drug therapy to treat his duodenal ulcer. Surgery to oversew the ulcer was performed following an acute deterioration in his condition. Prior to surgery, Mr Randall was treated with intravenous chlormethiazole (a sedative) for severe confusion and agitation; these were attributed to hepatic encephalopathy resulting from alcohol-induced liver cirrhosis. In the recent past, he had received treatment for problems of alcohol dependency and liver disease.

A key task for the medical staff is to ascertain which of Mr Randall's symptoms are indicative of underlying, chronic and *irrecoverable* pathology and which are attributable to acute, *recoverable* disease or to the side effects of drugs administered to him. This process involves the collection and interpretation of various forms of clinical data, and the gathering of opinions from other medical specialists. Since these activities are both spatially and temporally distributed, a cautious approach to the medical management of Mr Randall's condition is followed. This allows the information from the various sources to be assembled and debated. Treatment options are moulded on the basis of consensus opinion: some forms of treatment are continued in spite of doubts voiced by some of the medical personnel as to their overall efficacy. The following extract from the field notes, taken on days six and seven of Mr Randall's case, illustrate the interdependence of the various medical teams involved in his management and the difficult process of aligning their various interpretations of his condition. Mr Randall's sedation has been stopped for three days (although as we shall see below there is uncertainty among the intensive care staff as to the timescale of this), but he remains unresponsive apart from coughing when endotracheal suction is given:

(Day 6)
At 08:30 the senior registrar, last night's duty registrar and the new duty registrar arrive at Mr Randall's bed. (The registrar speaks extremely quietly to the SR, I cannot hear clearly what is being said.)

SR: 'He was very acidotic on Friday, is that better?'

The registrar picks up the medical notes file and starts to read the flow sheets with the blood results on in response to this question. All three doctors spend some time poring over the figures, and deduce that there is some improvement, since Friday.

Registrar 1: 'The physician has said that it may take a week for him to
   clear the heminevrin [a sedative given on the ward prior to surgery].'
SR: 'That long?' He frowns and says doubtfully: 'Well, we'll just have
   to carry on.'

He turns to the nurse (T) who has not been part of the conversation until now: 'How long has the sedation been off now?'
T: 'A few days – about 36 hours I think.'
SR: 'He's coughing and swallowing is he?'
T: 'Yes.'
SR: 'Oh, well, that's more than at the weekend.'

T and the doctors discuss whether or not his intravenous lines need changing, they decide that these need to be renewed. The medical staff leave with a view to returning later to do this.

I notice that the physiotherapists have arrived. One comes across to T: 'Is it OK if we come in here in a few minutes?' T nods. The surgical team arrive before the physios start treating Mr Randall. They are conspicuous because of their white coats. They briefly stop by Mr Randall's bed and ask about his wound. They move quickly to another patient when they are satisfied that the wound is not leaking undue amounts of fluid . . . Later in the morning, Consultant D arrives to assess Mr Randall. He listens to his chest briefly and to his abdomen. I note that Mr Randall is being both enterally and parenterally fed, and that he has a pyrexia now of 38°C. Consultant D writes in the notes that nothing has been cultured from the various samples sent to the bacteriology lab. and what his current antibiotic treatment is (flagyl and cefotaxime). He notes in the medical file that he is: 'slow to wake up – probably due to poor liver function and large amounts of sedation.' I note that Mr Randall's vasopressin [a drug for cardiac support] has been restarted. He is also receiving dopamine and bumetanide to support his renal function, and insulin to adjust hyperglycaemia.

(Day 7)
13:15. Report given in the coffee/staff room. Mr Randall has apparently deteriorated during the night. His temperature is now 39.2°C and he has developed a tachycardia and copious diarrhoea. His ventilation had to be adjusted during the night to cope with his tachyopnoea. The charge nurse giving the report, reports that the surgeons and consultant anaesthetists have agreed this morning that in view of his deterioration and the fact that he has not 'woken up' any more, that 'aggressive treatment' will be withdrawn. (Presumably referring to his drug therapy, although this is not made clear.) However this is not a final decision – they need to speak to both the consultant physician and to Mrs Randall

At 14:00 the consultant physician arrives to review Mr Randall. He goes behind the curtains with Consultant D and the senior registrar. Shortly afterwards he leaves, and the nurse, K, draws the curtains back. I go and ask her what the two consultants spoke about. She tells me that the physician agreed that Mr Randall's prognosis was very poor, but that in his opinion not enough time has elapsed to allow all traces of sedative to be excreted. He recommends waiting at least another 36–48 hours. He does agree however that if another body organ fails, then withdrawal of his drugs should take place at that point. K tells me that both consultants have discussed the possibility that Mr Randall may have had a 'cerebral catastrophe' but agree this cannot be confirmed, and that therefore treatment must be continued as it stands.

(From the field notes)

This extract illustrates the attempts made by the anaesthetic staff (who cover the day-to-day work of intensive care) to clarify the cause of Mr Randall's depressed consciousness. They attempt to rule out an acute, metabolic cause by scanning the available blood results for signs of improvement. When signs of an acute cause are not identified, they discuss other possible causes of unconsciousness and agree, apparently reluctantly, with an opinion given earlier by the admitting consultant physician: that sedatives administered prior to surgery for symptoms of alcohol withdrawal may still be affecting him. Similarly, the duty consultant comes to this conclusion when he examines Mr Randall later in the morning. Both the consultant and the junior medical staff attempt to pre-empt further acute changes in Mr Randall's condition by ensuring that the everyday practices of infection control and monitoring are diligently carried out – thus plans are made to renew intravenous catheters and results from the bacteriology laboratory are scanned in an attempt to locate the source of Mr Randall's temperature. The surgical team visit briefly and fulfil their responsibilities by assessing the condition of Mr Randall's laparotomy wound; they do not at this point discuss his overall condition with the other medical staff.

Mr Randall suffers a sudden deterioration in his condition during the night of day six and the early hours of day seven. His developing sepsis and renewed cardiovascular instability, together with his continued unconsciousness, lead to a tentative plan to start to withdraw the drug treatments given to him. The charge nurse describes how this plan is a result of discussion between the anaesthetic and surgical staff, and indicates that final confirmation of the proposal can only be made when the consultant physician has given his opinion. When the consultant physician arrives, he persists in his view that Mr Randall's neurological impairment may still be due to the lingering effects of sedation, rather than to an irreversible, rapidly progressing, chronic hepatic encephalopathy. He does, however, shift his position slightly by allowing for the possibility that a 'cerebral catastrophe' has occurred, although he stresses that this is impossible to confirm from available clinical data. While the exact parameters of 'improvement' or 'failure' are not discussed, thus creating an opportunity for further negotiation as to the interpretation of particular clinical signs, the consultant physician agrees with the proposal to withdraw drug treatment from Mr Randall if there is no neurological improvement over the next 48 hours or if further organ failure develops.

The discussion has so far focused on the impact of accounts of health history and quality of life on the interpretation of clinical data, the demarcation of pathology into 'recoverable' or 'irrecoverable' categories and the subsequent delimitation of medical action. In each of the case examples an indication has been given of the complexities and contextual features involved, and particular themes have recurred. These include the characteristic reproduction of the ill person as a list of physiological, medical-technical problems; the extensive range of clinical data that is available for analysis;

and the involvement of various medical specialists in the preliminary diagnostic process. I now examine these themes in more detail.

Legitimating technological knowledge

Anspach (1987) has suggested that the organization of work within the intensive care unit is such that the healthcare professionals rely on different sources of knowledge. Accordingly nursing staff make prognostic predictions on the basis of intuition, while medical staff predict on the basis of 'hard' technological data. My own study partially supports Anspach's observation, but suggests that experiential and intuitive knowledge is important for both groups of professionals, and that particular strategies are employed to ensure that information from this source of knowledge is aligned to the 'hard' technological data.

A major aspect of this is the role played by medical 'routine', which has the effect of 'prestructuring the pathological reality' (Berg 1992: 158). The routines that are examined here are the 'ward round' and the use of the medical notes. Both offer strategies for containing the element of risk involved in the management of a complex and rapidly changing situation in which many different parties are involved. An examination of the conversation between healthcare professionals during ward rounds demonstrates how different influences on data interpretation shift temporally *across* the course of an individual's illness and also spatially, according to the situational context – *who* was communicating with *whom* and *where*. In this way the concepts of 'probably dying' or 'probably recovering' are actively constructed. Further, medical and nursing staff use the vehicles of the formal ward round and the compilation of notes to collate and document the emergent technological data, and to align their working practices such that a sense of common purpose and respect is engendered.

The role of routine practices

Mrs Taylor was admitted to intensive care at Eastern hospital from the operating theatre following emergency surgery for perforation of the large bowel. She had been admitted to a surgical ward four days earlier and on admission to the surgical ward had also been diagnosed as suffering from pneumonia. Mrs Taylor had a history of chronic ill health, and had suffered two cerebrovascular accidents, a myocardial infarction, persistent atrial fibrillation and epilepsy. Her husband, Ernest, cared for her at home and attended to all her physical needs: lifting, feeding, dressing and bathing. Mr and Mrs Taylor had no children, their closest relatives were Mr Taylor's brother and his wife.

On day three of Mrs Taylor's intensive care treatment (the first day of observation) I note the duty registrar sitting at the table at the end of Mrs Taylor's bed reading her intensive care notes and then picking up her ward notes and leafing slowly through them. Having done this he gets up and examines Mrs Taylor; listening to her chest and checking the monitor that displays physiological data. He then returns to the table and writes down his findings in the intensive care notes. Mrs Taylor's nurse, J, seems annoyed because the registrar leaves Mrs Taylor's chest uncovered as he finishes his examination – J covers her up, and speaks to her, and starts to comb her hair. Mrs Taylor appears to be unconscious and makes no response to the nurse or to the doctor. Shortly after this, and while the registrar is still reading the notes, the 'nutrition team' arrives accompanied by the senior registrar to conduct their regular ward round:

> 11:00: *At the end of the bed the nutrition team has arrived and are quizzing the senior registrar and the registrar about Mrs Taylor's nutritional status and her past medical history. The notes are gone through again, and there is a prolonged discussion about her need for extra nutrition given that she was chronically ill before her admission, and was not fed prior to surgery. Several semi-humorous/black comments are made by the senior registrar and registrar during this discussion and they refer to her chances of recovery as: 'pissing in the wind'. Nonetheless great care is taken to analyse the figures of her biochemistry and haematology results and produce a prescription for total parenteral nutrition appropriate to the deficits 'seen' in the figures. Nurse J is not involved in this discussion except when there is a debate as to Mrs Taylor's normal weight and her height. (The SR presents Mrs Taylor as: 'just a poor old lady living at home being looked after by her husband', before giving a more 'medical' account of her history to the nutritionist.)*

> 13:00: *No activity around Mrs Taylor's bed, she lies motionless on her side. Sedated/ventilated. Oxygen down from 85 per cent to 80 per cent, having bouts of atrial fibrillation. At 13:45 the bacteriologists arrive and examine the results from her specimens sent on previous days. They point out that she has a positive sputum sample to coliform (the cause of her pneumonia) and check that she is on the correct antibiotic.*

>   (From the field notes, day 3)

What is visible here is an ordering and documentation of the clinical data collected on Mrs Taylor such that discrete medical actions, in this case the production of a prescription for intravenous feeding and appropriate antibiotics, can be organized. This excerpt illustrates the way in which medical action in intensive care becomes constructed as a series of closely focused tasks aimed at normalizing physiological data. The presence of the specialist teams – whose transient attention is directed at just one aspect of disordered physiology – enhances and lends authority to the process whereby the ill person is fragmented and reproduced (in various documents, prescriptions, results, and notes folders) as a series of potentially reversible physiological problems. Each of these has its own 'routinely' constructed plan of treatment and investigation. In this way, medical action is focused precisely: its range and extent limited to a clearly defined framework of options.

The comments from the intensive care doctors (the senior registrar and registrar) which re-frame their clinical activities as *'pissing in the wind'*, and the subject of their attentions as *'just a poor old lady'*, together with the co-existing nursing actions (the covering of Mrs Taylor's body from public view, the dressing of her hair, the verbal reassurance) seem, at first sight, to have the effect of de-stabilizing this whole process whereby medical action is legitimated and organized. The microscope of physiology is suddenly removed and 'Mrs Taylor' is seen in a different, diffuse, multi-dimensional context. Such scenes were visible both during the formal ward round presentations of Mrs Taylor's condition, and in the informal conversations of the intensive care staff. For example, in the afternoon of day three (a few hours after the round by the nutrition team responsible for dietary advice) the duty consultant conducts his round and betrays his own intuitive feelings about Mrs Taylor's overall prognosis. These threaten, briefly, to diverge sharply from the view informed by an analysis of clinical data; but the consultant deftly subsumes one to the other by means of his use of the notes, biochemistry results, and X-rays:

> 15:45 – Consultant B: 'She's not too bad, and yet, I don't know, I feel very uneasy about her.' He examines the notes and the X-rays, pointing out that her X-rays have improved but this has not been matched by clinical improvement, and the oxygen she is receiving cannot therefore be reduced. He looks through her blood results and points out a metabolic acidosis (often a sign of necrotic tissue somewhere), he says he suspects that her abdomen may be a focus of sepsis or necrosis and asks R (who has taken over from J) and the SR to keep a close 'eye' on her.
>
> (From the field notes, day 3)

This clash of perspectives is repeated over the course of the following days, even though there are some signs of improvement in Mrs Taylor's condition: there has been a reduction in the amounts of oxygen, sedation and inotropic drugs that she requires and some indications of improved neurological function. By the eighth day however, Mrs Taylor develops a temperature and her level of consciousness deteriorates. The surgical team are asked for an opinion and confirm that she may be suffering from renewed abdominal sepsis. Their terse entry in the notes reads: *'Continue present management, surgical intervention not appropriate.'* This referral to the surgical team demonstrates the way in which the intensive care ward rounds were situated within a context of on-going negotiations between the intensive care staff and the surgical team that had performed surgery on Mrs Taylor. These negotiations clarify their respective roles in her treatment, and ensure that the treatments given to Mrs Taylor by the intensive care staff are consistent with the surgeons' particular perspective regarding her chances of recovery.

The following day I join the consultant ward round as the intensive care staff are discussing Mrs Taylor's case. Consultant C (who is on duty that day) speaks to me:

> As I join the round Consultant C turns to me and says: 'Are you following this one?'
> Me: 'Yes.'
> Consultant C: 'Oh, she's a dead cert. A dead ringer.'
>
> (From the field notes, day 9)

This stark comment again threatens to undermine the ordered pursuit of individual physiological problems but, as in the previous example, his words are quickly absorbed and buffered by the rituals of the ward round, which involve the presentation of Mrs Taylor's case, the rereading of previous notes and the production of an ordered list of concerns:

> The duty registrar presents Mrs Taylor's case, telling Consultant C about the drainage of pus per rectum and the referral to the surgeons who are reluctant to operate. Consultant C: 'Let me see what they have written.' He takes the notes and reads the surgeon's entry from yesterday. While he does this the SR asks him: 'What should we do, with inotropes, if she becomes septic?'
>
> Consultant C: 'Let's go through everything and then we can make some decisions here'. They talk about her coliform infection (isolated in her sputum and wound) and about how concerned they have been about:
>
> (i) Her circulation – has she had a dvt [deep vein thrombosis]? Dosage of heparin?
> (ii) NG [naso-gastric] aspirate, which is heavily bile stained whether they try to feed her enterally or not.
>
> They suspect that (ii) is particularly significant and is related to an ongoing pelvic infection.
>
> (From the field notes, day 9)

Immediately after the production of this list, and before he responds to the request from the senior registrar to make a decision regarding the use of inotropic drugs, Consultant C enquires about Mrs Taylor's family situation. He is told about Mr Taylor's belief that the imminent 'new moon' will have a beneficial effect on his wife's health. The social context of the ward round allows for a communal expression of compassion for the older man and of embarrassment about his belief. In this way the threat of an alternative perception concerning Mrs Taylor is dealt with and the conditions re-created in which Consultant C can, (on the basis of the earlier decision by the surgeons that further surgery is inappropriate), conclude the problem of the inotropes:

Consultant C: 'What about her family?'

The senior registrar reports that Mrs Taylor's husband has had a 'bleak picture painted.' She recounts what she told him yesterday, and how she fears that he does not understand the situation clearly and how he seems to be putting his faith in 'the new moon' – there is some embarrassed laughter and murmurings of: 'poor old thing'.

Consultant C (thinking): 'I don't think we should start inotropes if she becomes septic.' He looks around the group.

Senior Registrar: 'I agree with that.'

Registrars 1 and 2 (seemingly to get practical details clear since they will be responsible for these) question the classification of inotropes: it is determined that dopamine may be used to encourage urine output, but not for 'drive' [cardiac function], similarly dobutamine.

Consultant C starts to write in the notes (I read this afterwards): 'This lady is not for aggressive treatment in the event of a re-occurrence of sepsis. Otherwise continue present treatment.'

(From the field notes, day 9)

As well as incorporating the intuitive feelings of the medical staff and the alternative perspective expressed by Mr Taylor, the ward round presents an opportunity for aligning the working practices of the medical and nursing staff. During the observational period the format of the ward round was altered to encourage co-operation between medical and nursing staff, and in recognition of the responsibilities of the 'primary nurse' for his or her patient.[5] I witnessed the anxieties of the nursing staff as they prepared for the ward rounds during the first few days of this new arrangement, and listened to the discussions between them about Mrs Taylor:

Handover from J to T and M. They discuss how she has slowly improved over the last three days. Mrs Taylor is sitting up in the bed. She has a face mask on and is following people with her eyes. Her breathing looks laboured. She has a nightgown on.

T: 'She's got a lovely smile, she smiles with her eyes.'

J: (whispering) 'I'm really getting fond of her now – mind you, that will make it harder [if she dies] – it's easier somehow if they're asleep and you don't get that connection with them.'

J explains that Mrs Taylor has been extubated. On the ward round yesterday it was decided that she should be aggressively weaned and given a chance to breath via a face mask before a tracheostomy was made . . . She was apparently extubated at 11:30 and has managed to speak once.

M: 'I don't think she looks good – I bet she doesn't manage for long.'

T: 'I think she looks OK – you must remember, what is she like normally?'

J explains the proposal put forward by Consultant A: trial of extubation, if she does not manage, reintubation and then percutaneous tracheostomy. During this period of uncertainty the heparin infusion (which she has been receiving for suspected deep vein thrombosis or pulmonary embolism has been turned off to minimize the risk of bleeding during the tracheostomy procedure).

S checks a blood gas, T takes it and looks at the figures. 'She's doing OK according to these.'

S: 'They're better than she looks.'

T is preparing for the nurse-led ward round – this is a new introduction since yesterday and means that from now on the Consultant ward round will be led by the nurse looking after the patient – he or she will present a summary and give an overview of the main issues/problems. T shows me the 'crib sheet' based on the various systems: cardiovascular, respiratory. She tells me: 'I was very nervous yesterday, but it went OK.'

14:30: T presents Mrs Taylor's case for the ward round, she gives a clear and comprehensive presentation including information about her 'normal' state: wheelchair bound, r. hemiplegia, smoker, degree of respiratory failure. At the end: Consultant B says to her: 'Well, you put my mates (the other doctors) to shame.' The doctors talk for a few minutes about how surprised they are that the nurses 'know so much' about the patients. (One of the 'G' grade sisters speaking to me about this later says: 'It's nice in a way but not in another, I mean, what did they think that we knew before?')

(From the field notes, day 16)

The format and agenda of the ward round is constructed carefully such that, although Mrs Taylor's case is presented by T (the primary nurse), her presentation becomes an exemplar of a proficient, medical report. The earlier references to emotion and appearance discussed in the nursing handover are omitted. T is congratulated on her performance by the consultant and the other doctors express their surprise at her 'knowledge' about Mrs Taylor. This style of participation in the ward round gives authority to T, and confirms her hierarchical position as a senior staff nurse *vis à vis* other nurses involved in caring for Mrs Taylor. After T's participation in the ward round on this occasion, I notice that Consultant B directs his questions about Mrs Taylor's condition to her, rather than to his junior medical staff. T uses this as an opportunity to voice her opinion that: '*I think if she stays here too long we're going to get too subjective about her.*' Consultant B responds with: '*I know what you mean but she has only just been extubated, she needs a day or so.*' After the ward round I ask T what she meant by 'becoming too subjective'. She explains that she feels that the medical treatment of Mrs Taylor is 'too focused':

> '*they are too concerned about her chest – how it is working – I think they ought to take a step back and think about what it is we are doing; you know, look at her as a whole, not just a pair of lungs to try get better – and anyway, how much better are we going to get her? I think that a tracheostomy would be just too invasive for her, and I think she should just be kept comfortable now.*'
>
> (From field notes, day 16)

T thus expresses her opinion that the close focus – on which medical action surrounding Mrs Taylor has so far been based – should be removed, allowing for a less 'subjective' approach as she nears the end of her life.

The following day (day 17), Mrs Taylor becomes increasingly unrousable. T looks after her during the course of the morning, but goes off duty before the consultant ward round in the afternoon. T hands Mrs Taylor's care over to C, and opines to C that Mrs Taylor has suffered a stroke and is no longer 'managing' (in a respiratory sense). C attempts to put across T's views in the ward round. The following extract from the field notes taken after the ward round illustrates the attempt made by the consultant to maintain the basis of medical action within the exclusive framework of tangible, clinical data (something which has been achieved successfully on all earlier occasions), rather than moving it to the more diffuse, experiential sphere occupied by T and C:

> *Consultant C and the senior registrar arrive to do their round, and staff nurse C starts to present Mrs Taylor's case. Consultant C obviously does not want to go over the same information as yesterday and interrupts her: 'OK, just tell us what is new C.'*

C seems a little flustered by this interruption, but gathers her thoughts:

C: *'Well, she was extubated yesterday and has managed so far on reasonable gases, but she is very much more sleepy and non-responsive, and is not able to cough at all now – we are having to do oropharyngeal suction.'*
Consultant C: *'Are you getting much up off her chest?'*
C: *'Yes, a lot of thick white secretions, and she has bronchial breathing on the left side.*
Consultant C: *'We still have not eradicated the pneumonia.'*
C: *'And T thinks that she may have had another stroke.'*
Consultant C: *'Let's have a look.'*

They go behind the curtains and he calls out loudly to Mrs Taylor. She does not respond. He examines her for focal neurological signs (which would indicate a specific lesion).

Consultant C: *'I'm not sure that she has had a stroke, I'm not sure what the problem is, one could go down a list of medical causes, you know: white blood cell count, magnesium, urea and electrolytes [he continues to list possible causes of drowsiness] but after excluding those -- well, you just don't know.' He turns to the SR: 'What do the surgeons think?'*
SR: *'They haven't seen her for 8 days.'*
Consultant C: *'8 days!'*
SR: *'Mr X -- I did 'phone them the other day, but they didn't come up.'*
Consultant C thinks.
SR: *'I think we should do a mini-tracheostomy and think about getting her to a ward now.'*
Consultant C: *'Yes, I think you are right.'*
SR: *'Should she be re-intubated again?'*
Consultant C: *'No, nor should she be readmitted to ITU. You'll have to get hold of the surgeons again and we'll have to speak to her husband. Is he here C?'*
C: *'Yes, he's outside.'*
Consultant C: *'OK, let's finish the round and then you (the SR) see him.'*
(From the field notes, day 17)

Thus Consultant C attempts to align what he can see, i.e. Mrs Taylor's unconscious state, with the biochemical data he has to hand. He attempts to confirm T's suspicions that Mrs Taylor has suffered a stroke by searching for clear neurological signs. He tries to quantify the extent of her respiratory failure by asking C specific questions. At the end of this process he has to come to the conclusion that, as far as a cause for Mrs Taylor's unconsciousness is concerned: *'you just don't know.'* At this point, the consultant makes reference to the surgeons and is seemingly surprised that they have not reviewed Mrs Taylor for 8 days. This expression of shock has the effect of re-affirming the shared responsibility of the surgical and anaesthetic teams in this case. For Consultant C, the fact that the surgical team seem to have already withdrawn attention from Mrs Taylor allows him to transfer his basis for action from that *allowed* by demonstrable clinical data to his own intuitive feelings about her condition. It is at this point that, for Consultant C, intensive care is no longer appropriate or meaningful in Mrs Taylor's case: he therefore recommends a further narrowing of the treatment options available, and asks the senior registrar to make arrangements to transfer her to a ward so that 'nature can take its course'.

Summary

In this chapter I have illustrated how diagnostic and prognostic certainty is achieved for critically ill individuals in intensive care. Case-study material illustrates the trajectory of four individuals, from the point of their admission to the point at which decisions are made that enable the complex process of limiting the delivery of intensive therapies. We have examined the formulation of accounts of 'health history' and 'quality of life', showing the critical impact of such accounts on the interpretation of clinical data. Further, the reproduction of the ill person as a series of 'acute' potentially treatable problems or of 'chronic' untreatable problems has been revealed as a means of delimiting 'intensive care'.

An illustration has also been given of the employment of the ward round and medical notes as 'routine' strategies for simultaneously legitimizing technological knowledge, for defusing other potentially conflicting perspectives, and for organizing and rationing the complicated, interspecialized nature of clinical work in intensive care. We see how:

> historical and examination data as well as medical criteria and disposal options are not 'givens' which unidirectionally lead the physician towards a disposal. The physician does not passively solve a puzzle with pre-set pieces: in articulating elements to the transformation, they are actively moulded and re-constructed. Furthermore it has been demonstrated how these elements intermix with other prevailing 'cross cutting systems of relevance' (Bosk 1979: 57) in medical practice.
>
> (Berg 1992: 168)

Hughes and Griffiths (1997: 589) describe such complex activities as the implicit 'ruling in' and 'ruling out' of therapeutic options: a process of micro-rationing that occurs at the clinical level and which remains largely invisible and inaccessible to 'lay' understanding. This chapter has shown that essentially elusive *social* and *subjective* criteria are involved in the planning of medical action in intensive care, but such criteria are represented, during interactional 'work', as a series of *technical* judgements. From here we can begin to focus more closely on the intersection between medical and nursing work in intensive care, shedding light on the way in which potentially contradictory perspectives of 'whole person work' and 'medical-technical work' are balanced, and conflict averted, during the care of critically ill people.

Notes

1 I have used the term 'quality of life' to refer to the everyday use of the term in intensive care rather than to any strict operational definition such as those contained in the extensive literature on quality of life measurement. The closest definition available to that employed in intensive care is the following: 'a polymorphous collage embracing a patient's level of productivity, the ability to function in daily life, the performance of social roles, intellectual capabilities, emotional stability and life satisfaction' (Dracup and Raffin 1989).
2 Since the completion of the fieldwork for this study, guidelines for admission to intensive care units in the UK have been published (Department of Health 1996) in an effort to avoid the situation of idiosyncratic decision making of this kind.
3 See Fox (1994) for a fascinating account of the use of the term 'fitness' by surgeons and anaesthetists.
4 The BMA guidelines (BMA 1999) which can be seen as a significant step forward in overcoming problems of bedside decision making, particularly with regard to the withdrawal and withholding of treatment, had not been published at the time these observations were made.
5 The ward round organization up until this time had been a 'presentation' given by the junior medical staff to the senior medical staff, with the occasional contribution from the nursing staff. The new arrangements gave the nurse at the bedside the responsibility of presenting the patient to the medical staff. This was done according to a set 'medical model' format. The medical staff were required to wait until the presentation was over, before discussing the relevant changes to treatment. This may have contributed to C's apparent 'fluster' when she is interrupted by Consultant B.

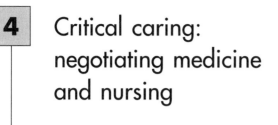

4 Critical caring: negotiating medicine and nursing

The ways in which relationships between nursing and medical staff evolve and are negotiated during the delivery and planning of treatment and care to critically ill patients are discussed in this chapter. Two areas are explored: the contrasting accounts given by doctors and nurses about their work, and the relationships between nurses and doctors during the delivery and planning of care and treatment.

In this way we see how medical work defines and encompasses nursing activity within intensive care. Indeed medicine is viewed as the context within which nursing operates and within which it must fashion its relationships with patients and their companions. However, nursing in intensive care will be shown to be dually constituted: first by the technical-medical work of medicine and second by strategies that incorporate 'whole person work' into this essentially depersonalized focus. Achieving and sustaining a balance between these constituents is a central feature of nursing work in intensive care. Medicine, in contrast, is characterized by attempts to ensure that 'body' is separated from 'person' and, further, that 'body' is deconstructed into a series of medical technical 'problems'. This studied fragmentation and depersonalization of 'body' ensures an efficient use of medical labour. It delineates clearly the sphere of medical responsibility and allows individual practitioners to manage and prioritize safely their complex burden of responsibility.

In the case-study data that follows we see how dissent emanating from the differing work perspectives held by doctors and nurses is rarely expressed openly; rather, disagreements are subverted during the processes of inter-professional interaction and negotiation. We start with a comparison of the accounts of 'work' given by medical and nursing staff.

Relationships between 'medicine' and 'nursing': a background

Current debates about the nature of nursing work highlight the emergence of a 'new' relationship between nurse and patient (Salvage 1990). The basis of this new relationship is seen as emotional exchange and the development of intimate knowledge about a patient by his or her nurse (Pearson 1988; Ersser and Tutton 1991; Swanson 1991). Caring 'for' in a practical, publicly visible, and task-oriented sense has been replaced in nursing discourse by the language of caring 'about' in an emotional, private, essentially invisible and person-centred sense (Savage 1995). Such concerns have been reflected by changes in the organization of nursing, which enhance continuity of care for patients by designation to them of a 'named' (Audit Commission 1991; Department of Health 1991; Hancock 1992) or 'primary' nurse (Pearson 1988; Wright 1990; Manthey 1992). Wider political and social forces emphasizing the professionalization of nursing, the accountability of nurses to their patients, and the patient as individualistic consumer have in turn focused attention on the 'quality' of the interpersonal relationship between nurse and patient (Bowers 1989; Audit Commission 1992; Savage 1995).

The recasting of the 'private' and the 'subjective' as a site of work in nursing (May 1992a,b) has brought to awareness a number of ambivalent features about 'nursing' and its relationship to medicine. Salvage (1995: 274) for example, makes the point that the apparent successes of nursing in refashioning the organization of care towards a more personalized model are undermined by: 'the central predicament of nursing as a woman's occupation in a man's world [and] the traditional marginalization of nursing by medicine and governments'.

One aspect of this 'traditional marginalization' has been the very invisibility of work that focuses on the formation of essentially private, intersubjective relationships. A number of empirical studies (Field 1989; Mackay 1993; Walby and Greenwell 1994) has demonstrated that the successful execution of such work is contingent on contextual and structural circumstances that are largely beyond the influence of nurses but in which doctors exert considerable control. For example, in a comparative study of the nursing care delivered to dying patients in various settings, Field (1989) demonstrated the difficulties facing nurses during the negotiation of the 'space' (1989: 122) required for those aspects of their work that are difficult for others to 'see' and for nurses themselves to articulate. Using terminology employed by Strauss *et al.* (1985), Field highlighted how the 'comfort' and 'sentimental' aspects of nursing work are *embedded within* the more visible activities of 'machine', 'safety' and 'articulation' work associated with the, essentially, medically controlled treatment of patients. As we saw in Chapter 1, in intensive care, the links between these various spheres of 'work' are intertwined particularly tightly (Cooper 1993, 1994; Walters 1994a,b, 1995). Intensive care nurses are presented with the opportunity of identifying themselves in relation to technological and diagnostic competency rather than to person-centred care, and it is this aspect of their role that is 'seen' by their medical colleagues:

> In ICU nurses have developed skills and accept responsibility for areas of treatment management that at one time would have been unquestionably within a medical domain. Consultants in ICU support the development of nursing skills, and set parameters within which nurses will decide on levels of sedation or assess change in ways that appear strikingly similar to making a diagnosis, but this is perceived as part of a process of providing care.
>
> (Walby and Greenwell 1994: 42)

The indissolubility of medical and nursing roles in intensive care presents a paradox for nurses: on the one hand their autonomy is increased and the respect they receive from doctors heightened because of their 'medical' knowledge and orientation. On the other hand, this legitimation of the medical aspects of their role threatens to undermine their ability to justify action on an alternative, essentially 'nursing' base. However, Svensson (1996) suggests that the complexity of, and overlap between, nursing and medical work in hospital areas like intensive care is such that relationships between doctors and nurses are no longer matters of dominance and hierarchy (Stein 1967; Freidson 1970) in which medicine constrains nursing overtly. Rather, negotiations are entered into during the interaction of clinical practice, which form and construct the very nature of nursing and of medicine:

> it is impossible in practice to draw any clear boundaries between the 'medical' and the 'nursing' fields . . . the field commonly termed medical questions is thus something constructed during interaction on the ward. Both the medical and nursing field are concepts created and modified by practice. How these areas are defined is largely an issue resolved through negotiations about the division of work on the ward.
>
> (Svensson 1996: 390)

Nursing and medical work in intensive care

Observation of clinical work around critically ill individuals in intensive care is confusing at first sight. Doctors and nurses work 'shoulder to shoulder' both giving directions and expressing opinions, beliefs and frustrations; they both engage in the many physical tasks involved in an individual's treatment. Closer examination, however, reveals that their roles are constituted quite differently. The medical staff have responsibility for initiating changes in treatment, for ordering investigations and for making summative diagnoses about the various complications that a patient may develop. The nursing staff, in contrast, have responsibility for ensuring that the various treatments are carried out safely and accurately and that the physiological data, on which treatments are based, are recorded and reported. These latter activities are performed alongside the physical acts more usually associated with 'nursing': washing, turning, clothing, redressing of wounds. Moreover, the delivery of physiological monitoring and bodily care by nurses is attended by the giving of reassurance to patients, and by judgements as to their need for comfort, sedatives or analgesia. The nursing staff also have primary responsibility for giving support, comfort and information to the ill person's companions; they do this in a primarily informal manner, incorporating such activities into their minute-by-minute work of attending to their patient. The medical staff, in contrast, come into contact with the ill person and their companions in a relatively sporadic way: they have equal responsibility for all the other patients in the unit, and have to 'spread' their attentions between them all.

Such differences in emphasis and responsibility between the two roles are visible in the interview data obtained from both nurses and doctors during the study. One of the intensive care registrars gave a vivid account of his perception of medical work in intensive care:

> Myself, I find intensive care rewarding simply because you read about physiology, pharmacology, this sort of thing and then you put it into action. You can be slightly depersonalized about it, you know, you're looking at figures rather than the patient, because the patient is ventilated or sedated and not talking to you, so that leaves them in a way without a personality. I mean you don't ever forget they're a patient, you're always trying to help them and at the end of the day you want to achieve an awake patient that has a personality and that's talking to you. But the discipline of the physiology side of things, trying to keep things in check, is something that I find good.
>
> (From retrospective interview, registrar, Western)

This doctor describes how he has to prioritize and problematize his work with critically ill patients in order to manage his responsibility for their often rapidly changing condition. He gives an insight into the stress he experiences in attempting to fulfil his responsibilities towards as many as six very ill patients at any one time, and the subsequent tensions he experiences in his relationships with the nursing staff, each of whom have primary responsibility for only one of those patients:

> At my level, at registrar grade, with the amount of experience I have got, it can be quite stressful because you know that you are going to be on call from 5 in the evening through until 9 the next morning . . . [and]

on very sick patients you literally do things every hour and every hour things could change. That's the idea – you respond to those things; you learn how to respond, but sometimes you feel as though you need some more back up . . . I mean if you know there are sick patients here, I personally find it quite daunting thinking 'oh, we're going to have a busy night', and that's why I prefer to get to the sickest patients first, see them first and call the seniors before it's too late and say: 'Right, these are the problems I've got, this is what I want to do, or this is what I think we should do' . . . You seek out potential problems and make a plan for avoiding them . . . If you've got six patients, you have six nurses each looking after one patient whereas you're one doctor looking after all six patients, and each of the nurses sees their patient as the priority whether they are the sickest or not. They interrupt you while you're dealing with something else and they don't realize that, you know, just talking to you while you're thinking about another problem breaks your concentration on that problem.

(From retrospective interview, registrar, Western)

In contrast to the organization of medical work (which was similar in both units), nursing work was structured very differently. In both units, one nurse would assume responsibility for the overall nursing care of each ill person and one nurse would care for one patient on a shift-by-shift basis. Similarly, the description of 'work' given by the nurses in both units was markedly different to the descriptions furnished by the medical staff. Nurses acknowledged the specialized, medically oriented aspects of intensive care nursing work, *but* they placed these discrete activities in the context of an emphasis upon the physically intimate and continuous nature of their involvement with patients as well as the process of building close relationships with patients' companions. The nurse interviewed below seems to imply that this close, involved character of her work enables her to, first, 'direct' the attention of medical staff towards the 'problems' that constituted *their* work and, second, to reach an overall assessment of the patient's 'best' interest and chances of recovery:

You look after, you do total patient care and I think we look after, I think nurses more or less co-ordinate the patient's care. We're there to nurse them . . . keep them nice and clean and tidy and respectable and make sure they get all the drugs that the doctors prescribe. But we're also there 24 hours a day so that we know when a patient's not responding appropriately, so that we can 'phone the doctors so that treatment can be done and investigations done . . . a lot of our work is I think prompting doctors without our telling them . . . They base their care on the observations that we've seen because we're there all the time with the patients . . . we try to guess what [patients] want out of the treatment and try to make sure that the treatment's appropriate for them . . . you're there to help the family through the patient's illness as well because it always affects the relatives when someone's in ITU.

(From retrospective interview, staff nurse, Eastern)

The emphasis in this extract on 'total patient care' involving many different activities was a characteristic feature of other accounts of work presented by nurses:

I feel that the nursing staff on ITU have the overall responsibility for everything that happens to the patient, be it being the general nursing care and looking after the patient's psychological and clinical well-being plus looking after the relatives and all the medical interventions that happen to the patient, you feel directly involved with [the patients].

(From retrospective interview, staff nurse, Eastern)

it's one of the few areas that you can give total patient care . . . I know it's an area where I can give the patients and relatives the best possible care . . . you see the person and you pride yourself on being able to provide a holistic approach to their care

(From retrospective interview, staff nurse, Western)

The multi-dimensional nature of nursing in intensive care and the repeated appeal to the discourses of 'holism' and 'total patient care' meant that nurses' perception of their patients was weighted away from the more 'detached' impersonal stance which the doctors attempted to occupy. Instead, nurses tended towards describing their patients as 'known' individuals, with particular, *personal* styles of response to treatment not dependent on 'hard' demonstrable, measurable data. This occurred even though many patients were unconscious and had never been 'known' as conscious beings to the nurses caring for them. Nurses thus achieved balance between the various constituents of their roles: they co-operated with the technical management of the patient's body and entered into the discourse of physiological response, but they also described the bodily response in terms that attributed subjectivity to the unconscious patient. In this way, the mechanization of nursing work was avoided and the demands placed on nurses to achieve interactive, intimate relationships with their patients were met. Chapter 7 looks more closely at how nurses attributed subjectivity to the apparently lifeless bodies of their patients in a discussion of 'nursing care only', taking up Lawler's point that for nurses to live up to the discourse of holism in contemporary nursing theory: 'One cannot simply nurse the body in the bed. One must do business with it as a person because nursing means being able to view the body and the person as inseparable' (1991: 34).

Containing conflict between nursing and medicine

The alignment of the intimate, interpersonal aspects of nursing work with the technical, medical demands of their role, in which they supported and co-operated with the treatment 'tasks' of the medical staff, resulted in a marked dissonance between the public performance of nurses' work and their private, informally expressed opinions about their labour. Although such dissonance was at times shared by the medical staff (as we saw in the account of 'Mrs Taylor' in the previous chapter), it was a more commonly observed feature among nurses. Further, the realization among nurses that medical staff were constrained by virtue of the demands of their 'work' to respond towards patients in ways that excluded any open acknowledgement of the more intuitive and experiential spheres of knowing, resulted in a 'cloaking' of conflict between the two groups.

In order to illustrate these points we will rejoin the case of Mrs Hall from Western Hospital, highlighted in the last chapter. A clear picture of the nature of medical work has emerged in which Mrs Hall is reproduced as a bundle of physiological characteristics. These are framed as 'problems'; each of which is individually addressed by the use of particular drug and treatment regimes and by referral to other specialists. A clear illustration of this tendency is the way in which Mrs Hall's illness is described to her daughter, Karen, by the registrar who had admitted her:

> I read the relatives' information sheet,[1] where the registrar from yesterday has carefully written what she said to Karen: she explained that Mrs Hall had improved since Wednesday night but that there were still a number of problems: 1) Respiratory infection and failure – X-ray showed old scarring. 2) Heart not pumping adequately. 3) Swollen liver because of back pressure from the heart. 4) Kidneys not working very well. All these problems were being treated by 1) ventilation, oxygen and suction. 2) By medicine to help the heart pump more effectively. 3) Sedation to keep her comfortable.
>
> Karen told that Mrs Hall's chances were 50–50.
>
> (From the field notes)

The doctor giving the information had indicated to me earlier that she had gained a sense of personal satisfaction and professional confidence from averting the near death of Mrs Hall in the Accident and Emergency department. She tells me how she is aware that Mrs Hall may not survive, but is pleased by her limited, cardiovascular improvement. Her 'work' seems to centre around viewing Mrs Hall as a challenge and an opportunity to learn. This orientation is validated when she receives praise from the intensive care consultant for doing 'a good job' during her initial assessment and treatment of Mrs Hall.

I became aware that the nurses looking after Mrs Hall had a very different perception of 'a good job'. It became clear that the nursing staff did not have the same level of confidence in the medical portrayal of the patient. They tended to be influenced less by the potential solubility of her individual physiological problems and more by the overall pessimism engendered by her age, frailness and the interactive nature of those physiological problems. These differing perceptions of 'doing a good job' reflect the ways in which nurses and doctors perceive the constitution of their roles and are illustrated clearly in the following extract. The notes were recorded on the second morning of my observation of this case:

> *At 7:45 the senior registrar arrives, he goes round briefly and checks the patients. He sits next to me at the nurses' station and I ask him how he thinks Mrs Hall is: 'Mrs Hall? – Oh, she's OK. Well, let's put it like this, she's better than she was on Wednesday night, and I think she'll be OK eventually.' The G grade sister who is also sitting at the station gazes at him in almost a derisive manner and explodes: 'Ha!' The senior registrar responds to this expletive lamely: 'Oh, well, maybe not. X doesn't agree with me.'*
>
> *Sister: 'She's got so many things wrong with her!'*
> *SR: 'That's true, but at least she's shown that she can put up her cardiac output to 6 litres from 4 yesterday – I know she's on noradrenaline but that is better.'*
>
> (From the field notes)

This exchange captures the different views of Mrs Hall held by the nursing and medical staff, and is further reflected during subsequent events around her bedside. For example, at lunch-time on the second day of observation, the registrar asks the staff nurses caring for Mrs Hall whether they feel that she can 'manage' with a reduction in her sedation with a view to 'weaning' her from the ventilator. One of the nurses expresses her unhappiness about this proposal, stressing how agitated she believes Mrs Hall will become. The implication is that the nurse sees her role as primarily one of promoting Mrs Hall's comfort, rather than one of colluding in what may be a futile attempt to wean her from ventilation. The doctor says, almost apologetically:

> *'Well, I think we have got to try – we'll wean the midazalom down slowly, get her onto SIMV and then CPAP [part ventilation, part spontaneous breathing modes]. If her gases go off we will have to re-sedate her.'*
>
> *She moves away, Staff Nurses 1 and 2 look resigned and unhappy. 1: 'She won't do; I'm sure of it. I think they ought to leave her a bit longer like this and get her chest a bit better. They know she's got a chest infection (Staph. aureus has been grown from her sputum). She*

looks comfortable now as well . . . But just because she might get agitated is no reason not to try her off – she's going to have to be weaned I know that.'

(From the field notes)

In this short exchange it is possible to discern elements of sympathy between the staff nurses and the registrar. It appears that the doctor has a brief to engage in a particular 'routine' course of action: a reduction of sedation with a view to reducing mechanical ventilation. Her response to the staff nurses' anxiety reveals that she shares their view, but is constrained by the nature of her work such that she cannot use their opinions as a basis for action. The subsequent discussion between Staff Nurses 1 and 2 (summarized above) in which they acknowledge that Mrs Hall will 'have to be weaned' confirms the pre-eminence of the medical perspective and effectively removes the threat of their alternative view.

The following day (day three of observation), a similar problem reoccurs. On this occasion, the threat to the medical perspective on Mrs Hall is expressed more sharply, but is again effectively subverted by the actions of the nurses themselves. Mrs Hall's sedation has been stopped completely and, because she has still not made any attempts to breath spontaneously, a different drug has been administered in an attempt to reverse the action of the drugs used to sedate her. The unhappiness of Staff Nurses 1 and 2 observed the previous day is mirrored on this occasion by the expressed feelings of another nurse who is looking after Mrs Hall. I summarize my impressions of Mrs Hall in the field notes as follows:

Arrived to update on Mrs Hall. She is lying quietly but her eyes are moving rapidly under her eyelids and she occasionally moves her arms weakly. Staff Nurse 3 is looking after her, apparently the midazalom has been stopped but she has not 'woken up'; she has been given some flumazinil [a stimulant] to try to reverse the sedation – and she has moved all four limbs to command. However she is needing more oxygen to maintain her blood gases and her urine output is decreasing dramatically. She is now on an infusion of frusemide and her infusion of noradrenaline has been doubled in an attempt to increase her blood pressure but with no effect. Consultant 1 has now written in her notes that: 'dialysis would be inappropriate given her age and condition.'

(From the field notes)

Staff Nurse 3 is almost aggressive in her criticism of the medical management of Mrs Hall and attempts to gain support for her point of view from the charge-nurse and from the physiotherapist:

I ask Staff Nurse 3 how she thinks she is: 'Well – I'm sorry – it's swearing, I think she is fucked – and if I were her family I wouldn't be very happy about all we are doing. She's not even sedated – in fact they are trying to reverse her sedation with flumazanil. I'd want to be right out of it if I were her and in a similar state. But then I work here. I get the impression that her family think that we're all trying our best to get Nana better – maybe Karen is a bit ambivalent, but she's the only one. When people get to this sort of age I think they should be allowed to die peacefully – I really don't think we should be doing all this.'

Slightly later the physio arrives and asks Staff Nurse 3 how Mrs Hall is. Staff Nurse 3 explains about the sedation being left off and how her secretions which were thick and yellow yesterday seem to have dried up. 'How many times have we seen patients like this?' Staff Nurse 3 says: 'I think Consultant 1 is on an "everybody's going to live" streak.' The charge-nurse who is listening to the conversation agrees: 'I think you're right there.'

Physio: 'Have they said not to treat her?'
Staff Nurse 3: (sarcastically) 'No!'

(From the field notes)

Here we witness clear dissent from the nurse, who is concerned because Mrs Hall has been left unsedated in spite of the deterioration in her condition, which has necessitated the consultant's written note to the effect that dialysis treatment would be 'inappropriate'. Again this seems to stem from the differing work orientations of the medical and nursing staff – the medical staff are in pursuit of a treatable cause for her illness and wish to try all avenues of therapy, before feeling justified in calling a stop. To give sedation at this point – when many acute treatments are still being given – would signal that death was inevitable. The nurse feels concern for Mrs Hall's level of comfort and is scathing about the 'optimism' of the medical staff, especially as the continued treatment of Mrs Hall has now been circumscribed by the written note excluding dialysis as an option of therapy. She only expresses this dissent to myself, the physiotherapist and to her more senior nursing colleague, however, and then continues to attend to the medically framed tasks of helping with physiotherapy and checking observations. The anger of this staff nurse may be an expression of the discomfort she feels in having to continue with such tasks, in the face of what she recognizes to be – but is powerless to act on – the inevitable death of Mrs Hall.

By the afternoon the feelings of the staff nurse are borne out by the continuing deterioration of Mrs Hall. The senior registrar and the consultant agree at this point that:

(1) *There would be no active intervention re. renal failure.*
(2) *Glucose and insulin would be tried to lower her high potassium.*
(3) *The gravity of her condition should be discussed with her relatives.*
(4) *She should not be actively resuscitated.*

(From the medical notes)

There is a mixture here of continuation of some treatments – glucose and insulin, for example – but a reiteration of the decision not to give renal support is added to by a decision not to resuscitate her in the event of a cardiac arrest. That afternoon the senior registrar speaks to her family. In his written summary of the interview he makes a reference to the coroner – implying the certainty of death – but he falls short of recommending a withdrawal of treatment. He instead proposes that the 'status quo' is preserved and a decision delayed until the following day. The senior registrar thus places Mrs Hall's condition firmly within the established, medically acute, curative framework, and effectively disallows either an open recognition of 'dying', or the production of a prospective, multi-disciplinary plan to 'manage' that dying:

> *It was explained that despite the current maximal therapy that her kidneys and liver were failing. Outlook bleak. Renal support would not cure her. Treatment so far has been supportive for each part of her illness and no diagnosis of underlying causes. (No mention of need to refer to coroner.) Plan: keep treatment ISQ. May deteriorate rapidly – no benefit in resuscitating. May start drugs to keep her comfortable if needed. Review tomorrow and repeat discussion with the possibility of withdrawal.*
>
> (From the relatives' information sheet)

Summary

This chapter has delineated the constitution of medicine and nursing in intensive care, showing how nurses and doctors perceive their roles and then how those roles are enacted during the processes of care delivery. It has been suggested that a 'medical' interpretation of 'the patient', involving a discrete, problem-solving deconstruction of that individual, is supported by the co-operation of the nursing staff. This is in spite of a comparatively high degree of autonomy and the 'total care' orientation of the nurses, which compels them to reproduce the patient as a 'known', rather than depersonalized, entity. The co-operation of the nursing staff and their attention to the medically framed aspects of their role effectively subverts conflict between the professions: conflict that is expressed by nurses about medical treatment of those patients whom they believe to be dying is done so obliquely, rather than openly. I have suggested that this subversion of conflict is possible because of a realization that the medical staff are effectively constrained against basing their action on any footing other than the 'technological'; and that frequently the 'technological' measurement of dying lags far behind the consensus recognition of that state as a 'common-sense' fact. Chapter 6 examines this issue of potentially divergent dying trajectories with regard to the construction of non-treatment decisions by medical staff.

Contradictions produced within intensive care nursing as a result of the mismatch between the discourse of 'total care' and the demands of technical-medical problematization become particularly visible as critically ill patients move closer to death. Chapter 7 addresses more closely the ways in which such contradictions are managed by nurses and examines the concept of 'nursing care only': a term employed frequently to describe the care of patients who are no longer receiving curative medical treatment and who are expected to die within a short period of time.

The next chapter explores the extent to which patients' companions are involved in the process of treatment planning. The emphasis here is on the disclosure of diagnostic information to companions and the various ways in which they use and interpret such information.

Note

1 The relatives' information sheet was a means of recording details of what had been said during interviews between medical staff and relatives. It was used on both units.

5 A primary need examined: the disclosure of information to patients' companions

The issue of 'awareness contexts' (Glaser and Strauss 1965) and the disclosure of bad news has been a recurring theme in studies concerning the care of dying people and their companions over more than three decades. The usual focus of such work has been an analysis of the most appropriate ways in which news about poor prognoses or imminent dying can be given, and an examination of the negative consequences of 'closed awareness'. Implicit in the wealth of practical advice that has followed Glaser and Strauss is the assumption that knowledge or awareness endows people with the ability to play an active and fairly equal part with clinical staff in the decision-making process regarding the direction and level of future treatment whether for themselves, or for others (see, for example, Buckman 1992). At the heart of this assumption is a concern to examine ways in which 'autonomy' can be enhanced at the end of life, whether by seriously ill people themselves or, in those circumstances when they are unable to speak for themselves, by their close companions as 'proxy'.

This chapter examines some of the interactional intricacies involved in 'disclosure' and shows how difficult it is for staff to manage the process of giving information to companions in the face of their extreme distress. It will be seen how barriers between companions and staff can emerge because of the 'partial' knowledge accessed by staff of the wider history and social context of illness. It will also be seen how 'participation' in decision making is not a central aim of clinicians in intensive care: rather attempts are made to bring companions to a point where they will agree with decisions that have *already been* taken. In so doing, however, the conditions sometimes arise in which companions are able to exert influence over the direction and speed of the unfolding treatment trajectory.

Autonomy and 'best interests'

The issue of autonomy has become pre-eminent in discussions about end-of-life care, although it is in fact only one of the four key principles of bioethics, the others being beneficence, non-maleficence, and justice. Autonomy, on which the legal right of informed consent is based, is the capacity for self-determination and choice, free both from exterior compulsion or internal impairment (Pabst-Battin 1994). As Kelner notes (1995: 537), there is a pervasive belief not only that the exercise of autonomy is *possible*, but also that individuals have the *right* to act autonomously and make decisions about different options concerning their care. A fundamental challenge to the autonomist position is the argument that the exercise of autonomy is not possible. In this argument, constraints of a cultural, social, and clinical nature are identified as hampering free individual choice to such an extent that it becomes impossible to speak of independent choice.

The principle of autonomy is widely used to guide the policies and law surrounding end-of-life decision making (even though there is considerable evidence that clinical practice at the end of life is not always predicated on known patient preferences (Principal Investigators for the SUPPORT Project 1995)). For people not able to exert or express autonomy, there has been an increased emphasis on anticipatory treatment directions in the form of 'living wills' and 'advanced directives'. These have acquired undisputed legal status in the US, Canada, and Australia and have been a central, although more contested, issue in end-of-life deliberations in the UK (House of Lords' Select Committee on Medical Ethics 1994; Law Commission for England and Wales 1995; BMA 1999). Courts in the US, Canada and Australia have taken the view that neither incapacity, nor failure to have completed an advanced directive or living will, strike out an individual's right to autonomy. The task in this interpretation of the autonomy principle becomes one of ascertaining what that individual *would have wanted* given the particular configuration of circumstances in which they are now placed. To this end, 'proxy' decision makers, often family members, are recognized as being able to exercise the right of autonomy on behalf of another.

In the UK, proxy decision making of this type has not been favoured. This is partly a historical development, and partly a response to the recognition of a potential lack of correspondence between 'proxy' views and those of the person the proxy represents. Instead, a 'best interests' approach has been favoured, with clinicians usually being given the responsibility for the identification of those interests (Howse 1998). Those who favour the best interests stance point to the problematic status of choices or preferences, expressed by a person when well, to the later situation of their grave illness in which they are no longer able to confirm such expressions. A central issue here is what constitutes 'personhood' and the extent to which the essence of personhood and preferences change during the course of the bodily deterioration associated with illness (Roth 1996).

Clearly there is an overlap here, since both the autonomist and best interests deliberations involve careful examination, usually by means of discussion between family members and clinicians, of what the individual in question might have chosen for themselves. Further, in the UK it is required that patients' previously expressed wishes are included in best interest deliberations (BMA 1999). The major difference is in the location of the balance of power. In the proxy decision-maker scenario this is weighted towards the patient's family member or other appointed proxy. In the 'best interests' scenario, the balance of power is weighted towards the clinicians, who are accorded the right to act paternalistically *if* they see fit.

Information and knowledge in intensive care: the process examined

Jones *et al.* (1991) in an article on social support in intensive care, summarize the traumatic impact that an individual's critical illness can have on close relatives and companions:

> the very nature of Intensive Care brings a separation both physically and emotionally of the patient from their normal social support network. The care of the patient is taken over so completely that often *all sense of control* is lost by both patients and their relatives. It is recognized that events are perceived as stressful when they are not within the control of the recipient.
>
> (Jones *et al.* 1991: 67, my emphasis)

From this statement, Jones and colleagues seem to imply that a 'sense of control' may be regained if the ill person's companions are involved in the process of care and treatment surrounding them. The intensive care nursing literature suggests that the primary 'needs' of companions in intensive care are honesty, information, hope and emotional support (Molter 1979; Manley 1988; Coulter 1989; Youll 1989; Wilkinson 1995). Of these interrelated needs, the receipt of 'information' has been highlighted as of particular importance, both in relieving initial acute anxiety and in the later emergence of a sense of 'control' and empowerment. Coulter (1989), in an interview-based study of the relatives of intensive care patients, found that they referred to 'knowledge' rather than 'information'. She describes how 'knowledge' is important in helping individuals 'make sense' of critical illness and in giving a sense that the intensive care staff 'care' about the ill person. Leske (1992), in a detailed study of an individual case, describes how the woman in her study experienced feelings of 'overwhelming powerlessness' and of 'lack of control' during the early days of her husband's illness. The 'need to know' was described by this individual as of primary importance in relieving these feelings: 'suddenly I had a lot of questions which I wanted answered, but everyone had disappeared. I asked the nurse to come into the room. I picked up the sheets. I wanted to look. I had to know what I was dealing with . . . When I had my questions answered it was suddenly very calming.' (Leske 1992: 393).

The theme of 'control' recurs in other studies that focus on companions' experience of critical illness (Hall and Hall 1994; Tilden *et al.* 1995; Furukawa 1996; Fulbrook *et al.* 1999a,b,c). For example, in a retrospective survey of 32 companions of individuals who had died following a withdrawal of medical treatment, Tilden *et al.* (1995) noted that the majority of their respondents recalled the way in which they developed a sense of empowerment and inclusion following communications between themselves and the healthcare staff. The most helpful style of communication was that described as 'timely, unhurried, honest, (and) compassionate' (Tilden *et al.* 1995: 636). Indeed, respondents in this study described themselves repeatedly as 'starving' or 'hungry' for information.

The relationship between the provision of information and the emergence of any sense on the part of companions of being able to influence or 'control' events around critically ill people is not, however, straightforward. The delivery of information may in itself be fraught with problems concerning the 'mismatch' of perceptions between healthcare staff and companions over whether the individual is 'getting worse or getting better' (Degner and Beaton 1987). One of the staff nurses in my own study described the difficulties that this can cause, talking about her involvement with the family of a severely head-injured man who was making involuntary movements indicating a severe brain injury:

> any movement that he made whether it was a decerebrate movement which wasn't an appropriate movement, or not, they were thinking that was a good sign and trying to convince them it wasn't necessarily a good sign was very hard and you felt like the bad guy, . . . seeing the family I was trying to enforce that he wasn't making any positive progress. He was in fact not doing very well at all . . . eventually they came round to that idea and accepted it.
>
> (From retrospective interview)

One aspect of this problem is the mirage of the potential 'miracle cure' (Harvey 1996), which may be maintained by patients' companions during the ordeal of grief that so often accompanies critical illness. In such situations, the sight of technological 'life-support' equipment obscures impending death, *even when* there have been repeated warnings and explanations about the likely outcome of the illness.

Another problematic aspect in the delivery of information is the access of the intensive care staff to knowledge about the broader context of their patient's illness. They may not, for example, be aware of the extent to which companions have developed a *distrust* of health professionals: such distrust may have emerged from earlier experiences relating to the onset of the patient's illness and may have a fundamental impact on the character of the relationship between themselves and the intensive care staff. Conversely, an appreciation may be lacking of the companions' perceptions and expectations regarding the patient's illness: repeated warnings of a poor prognosis become inappropriate when an acute illness follows years of severe, disabling chronic illness in which death has been both expected and prepared for by people close to the patient.

In this study, the delivery of information to companions was seen as a major aspect of their role by both nursing and medical staff. The nursing staff tried to interweave the delivery of information to companions into the ongoing care of their patients: thus they would frequently keep up a running commentary to the patient's companions of what they were doing. One nurse described very eloquently her feelings about the relationship between the support of companions and her everyday nursing work. This involves not only 'talking' but also showing in a practical way that the ill person is being cared for:

> Sometimes they watch you do things...Just that in a way is enough...I think either being there doing, or being there not doing, being there sitting and talking to them, just being there
> (From retrospective interview, Staff Nurse, Western)

Nurses recognized, however, that some people found it too stressful to remain by the bedside for long periods of time. On these occasions they would try to spend time away from the unit talking with companions, but this could create difficulties for the delivery of patient care. One of the nurses described the difficulties of looking after a critically ill man at the same time as giving the support and information that his wife appeared to crave:

> *she's calm but reluctant to spend time on the unit. She seems to want to talk – I wish she would sit in here with him more because then we would be able to chat to her, at the same time as looking after him. As it is she spends a few minutes here and then goes out again. I've been out several times and spent a few minutes with her, but then I have to get back to the bedside.*
> (From the field notes)

Other nurses reported similar feelings of being 'torn' between the needs of companions for information and support and the demands of patient-focused work:

> because we are looking after critically ill people who need an awful lot of your time and it's very difficult to divide that time between them

and the family, trying to prioritize. I often put myself in their shoes – I'd want to be involved and I'd want somebody to sit with me and keep me up to date besides . . . I think you feel guilty because you can't give them 100 per cent.

(From retrospective interview, Staff Nurse, Eastern)

The medical staff had a much more formal relationship with companions than the nurses. They were expected to give 'formal updates' on the condition of the ill person and they did this away from the bedside in a designated interview room, with a member of the nursing staff in attendance. One of the consultant medical staff described how he perceived the relationship between the release of 'gradual' information by the nursing staff and the more 'telling all' information delivered by the medical staff. His comments about the role of information giving are supportive of Anspach's (1987) thesis of 'prognostic slanting' in which clinicians 'prepare the ground' for future decision-making scenarios:

I always try to say to the family that first of all we will be very honest with them and I say two things: that we believe the philosophy is to treat or not to treat patients. There's no half-way house and while we believe there is a slender chance of reasonable success . . . we will try very hard . . . equally I say to them that should we reach the point at which we feel the treatment is no longer appropriate we will tell them . . . I think the other aspect is the much more gradual thing that the nursing staff do. This is not a big thing about sitting in a room and telling all, it's actually about talking to them: talking to them about the ventilation, the oxygen. Telling them that the urine isn't so good -- This is a gradual process and it's often in this time period that relatives are coming to the conclusion in their own mind that -- they're not getting better.

(From retrospective interview, Consultant B, Eastern)

Both nursing and medical staff portrayed their role in giving information as a means of enabling companions to adjust to the likelihood of death and as a means of facilitating the preliminary grieving process. The following extract from an interview illustrates this point. It refers to the wife of a man who had suffered a severe head injury:

JS: One of the things that I thought you seemed concerned about [during observation] was that she was oscillating between the pessimistic and the optimistic. Why do you think that was so?

Staff Nurse: That she was veering towards the pessimistic?

JS: Yes; and at one point you were saying to her, you know, you mustn't get your hopes up too much, I'm paraphrasing, but that was the general picture that I got?

Staff Nurse: I think that was, er, I suppose I knew that he wasn't going to survive, or at least was unlikely to. You know after the first 24 hours and no improvement had been made, you just know the way things are likely to go, and you want to prepare people. You don't want it to be a huge shock to them.

(From retrospective interview, Staff Nurse, Eastern)

Data from two case studies illustrates the role of the healthcare staff in imparting information to companions and highlights some of the problematic issues that are involved during this process. The first case illustrates some of the problems experienced by the healthcare staff in dealing with 'Mrs Oldham', the wife of the man referred to above. The second example explores the issue of 'mismatches' of interpretation and understanding by looking at the response of the healthcare staff to the wife (Mary) of an ill man (John).

The role of 'trust' in information giving: Mr Oldham's case

Mr Oldham was a 55-year-old man who was admitted to the Eastern intensive care unit with acute pancreatitis, which had caused respiratory failure. He died 15 days after admission. His next of kin was his wife. Ten days observation was completed in this case.

When I first meet Mrs Oldham, I observe that she seems to prefer to sit in the waiting room away from her husband. She explains that this is because she finds it too stressful to remain at the bedside for more than very brief periods. In this way she highlights the importance of being not only able to trust the nurses looking after her husband, but also rely on them to provide her with the information necessary for her to understand what is happening to him:

'I like to know and understand what is happening and why. I know I'm a pain but I'm always asking. S and J have been so good – I remember them because they are the nurses I've seen most of – they explain everything to me so I feel I can sit out here and leave them to get on with it.'

(From field notes)

However, on subsequent days the healthcare staff report their problems in attempting to meet Mrs Oldham's expressed need for information:

S asks J how Mrs Oldham has been – they discuss the difficulties of giving her 'what she wants' which they see as only 'good news'. J reports how Mrs Oldham has said that she does not like the registrar (who gave her detailed information last night and warned her that Mr Oldham is still very ill with an uncertain prognosis). J tells me that: 'I don't quite know how to pitch it with her – she says she wants to know everything, but when you start to tell her things she often says: 'OK – that's enough, that's enough' – as if she doesn't really want to know.'

(From field notes)

Mrs Oldham gradually attempts to replace her occasional physical presence by telephone contact. This is perceived as problematic and irksome on several occasions. For example, she is perceived as overstepping her remit as 'relative' in the following extract:

At 10:00 A is helping with another patient and the 'phone rings. It is Mrs Oldham. H takes the call. On her return A wants to know what has been said. H: 'I just told her that he was stable – she knows I'm not his main nurse, I told her you were on A and she said: 'Why's that?' and: 'I don't know her.' I said, well we're a bit short today – she said: 'Why are you short? Aren't there enough nurses?' So I said it's just that we are a bit busy today.

A: 'She's not a bloody nurse manager – it's none of her business.'

(From field notes)

In the following extract a tentative relationship is established between Mrs Oldham and D, a nurse with whom she has not previously had contact.

At 15:30 the 'phone rings –[1] another nurse answers it and calls D: 'it's about your chap.' D comes to the 'phone: 'Hello, it's staff nurse speaking. Oh, hello Mrs Oldham, – J told me that you were here this morning, is that right? Well there hasn't been any change – his blood pressure and heart rate are stable right now – He's on 85 per cent oxygen – Yes, a little lower, but still very high. Yes . . . I know . . . it's been up and down a bit. My name? [She gives her name] I don't think you've met me before – I haven't looked after Mr Oldham before. (There is a long pause while Mrs Oldham speaks) . . . That's quite understandable, you're bound to have days like that . . . have you anyone with you at the moment? . . . 'phone whenever you wish – no, no, you're no trouble at all.' D (to me at the end of this call): 'Poor woman – she was crying and she says she can't handle it at all today.'

(From field notes)

D is not, however, able to continue the promised relationship later in the evening because of the heavy demands of looking after Mr Oldham. She tries to make amends the following day by sitting and talking with Mrs Oldham but is still constantly aware of her need to attend to Mr Oldham:

Mrs Oldham apparently 'phoned twice more in the evening – D told me that she couldn't get to the 'phone because of all the things she had to do for Mr Oldham and that she therefore sent messages: 'No change since you spoke to me last'. The night staff nurse who then spoke to Mrs Oldham later reported that Mrs Oldham had been upset that D had not spoken or at least called her back. D: 'I just did not have the time – the trouble is that sometimes the relatives need you as much as the patient does, but you can't give them what they need – I sat with her this morning and had quite a long talk, but it was to some extent clock watching – you know what it's like – that infusion's due through or whatever – all those things to think about that must be kept track of.'

(From field notes)

Mrs Oldham describes to me how she cannot be present physically because of her mental strain. Her telephone calls thus assume a special importance, as it is the only way to build a mental picture of what is happening to her husband. The information that she is given is not however, in her view, reliable; this disturbs her sense of fragile equilibrium tipping the balance of power still further away from her:

'Well, it's been doing my head in being here so I've not been here very much – I've been in contact over the 'phone – the trouble is that I get told different things and that throws me out – for instance A told me yesterday that they'd had trouble with his blood sugars, but when I asked today I was told that they're not really a problem. Also I expected J to be on the night shift and it wasn't it was S. Well, that's OK, but it throws me. I like to know who is looking after him because then I can picture them at the bed.'

(From field notes)

Even when she is present physically she is unable to take part in the information exchange process – she does not speak the language and is not invited to proffer her opinion. This does not prevent her from trying to listen and understand what is being said:

Consultant C's ward round starts. Consultant C, the SR and Registrar, J and H present. They stand at the end of the bed. Mrs Oldham remains seated and looks very anxious, trying to listen. Consultant C smiles at her – 'We're not doing anything to worry about; we'll tell you later in ordinary language what we think.' Mrs Oldham (slightly sharply) 'I'm not worried – I'm listening to you all'.

(From field notes)

We see here the difficult process of forging trusting relationships between staff and companions. The process of achieving an appropriate level and style of information disclosure to the profoundly anxious Mrs Oldham was profoundly problematic, with particular difficulties associated with interpreting, or 'reading' exactly what it was that Mrs Oldham required to meet her apparent demands for 'full information'. The nursing staff struggled to maintain consistency in their approach to Mrs Oldham in the face of what they perceived to be rather inexplicable, paradoxical behaviour and in the context of the heavy demands of attending to Mr Oldham.

We now turn to an example that highlights how difficult it can be for information to be exchanged in the face of completely different understandings about the situation at hand. Here the efforts of the intensive care staff to prepare a wife for her husband's death fall apparently on deaf ears and it becomes clear that such preparatory activity was regarded as utterly irrelevant by the person to whom it was directed.

A mismatch of perception: John's case

John Smith was a 55-year-old man who had been chronically ill for many years. He was admitted to Eastern intensive care unit for specialist assessment of gastro-intestinal bleeding, liver and lung disease. He died after 10 days, following a withdrawal of drug treatment. His wife was his next of kin. Five days observation were completed in this case.

Throughout the period of observation here, John's wife, Mary, exhibited an apparent lack of distress and seemed unwilling to spend too long at the hospital. This worried the intensive care staff, who discussed her behaviour frequently, attributing it to lack of understanding and disbelief engendered by grief, rather than to any other cause. I noted similarly with some surprise on the first day of observation that Mary did not talk about her husband's acute illness to the extent that I expected. She told me instead details about the way in which her family's life has been affected during the years of John's chronic illness and about their financial difficulties. She did not, unlike other people I had spoken to, speak at any length about her hopes and fears for his recovery. She appeared instead to keep such feelings at bay, only occasionally showing her distress. In the morning of the second day of observation I am asked by A, the nurse looking after John, to go and bring Mary and her daughter from the waiting room. John's condition is very unstable:

She [Mary] tells me that they have not seen him yet and lets me take them into the unit. There is still a lot of activity around the bed, Nurse A acknowledges them with a nod of her head and rushes past to the drug cupboard. I try to make space around the bed so that they can sit down, and go to find chairs. Mary flushes red with distress when she sees her husband and sits and clasps his hand. He looks desperately ill

– frail, jaundiced, unconscious, surrounded by machinery. He is partly covered by a sheet but otherwise naked. Her daughter reaches for some tissues to give to her. A comes back – she reaches down and touches Mary's shoulder and then squats down to talk to her. The 'phone rings and A is called away to answer the enquiry – it is the other daughter that I met yesterday. A calls Mary to talk to her and we can hear her saying: 'He is not so well today, his blood pressure is very low.' When she finishes Mary goes back to the bed and sits down again, she is still very red faced. A is now sitting at the end of the bed working on the computer and the senior registrar is sitting next to her writing in the medical notes.

(From the field notes)

While Mary's distress is obvious at this point, by the time she has a formal interview with Consultant C a few hours later she has regained her composure, and seems keen to get the interview over so that she and her daughter can leave to get home. Nurse R has taken over from Nurse A now. The following extract from the field notes, written after that interview, reveals the efforts that Consultant C makes to explain John's condition, and to check any feelings of optimism that Mary may have. Mary seems to reject his efforts and brings the interview to a close. Consultant C is puzzled and seems slightly 'put out' by her reaction:

Suddenly, Consultant C says: 'Right, let's talk to the family.' Nurse R and he move towards the door (I have previously asked Mary if I can be present during this interview and she has agreed), I ask them if I may accompany them – 'Oh, yes, no problem.'

Mary stands up as we all go through into the waiting area: 'I'm glad you've come, we've got to go and get our bus soon.' We all go through to the interview room. Consultant C struggles to explain what they have been doing.

Mary: 'I noticed that his blood pressure is a wee bit better now?'
Consultant C: 'Well, yes, that's because of some different fluids that we have given him – but you know, as I've already told you, he is extremely ill and the chances of him surviving are very slim – having said that, he has improved very slightly over the last hour or so, but you mustn't get your hopes up.'
Mary: (Brightly) 'Well, he's not any worse then, we must be thankful for that.'
Consultant C: 'No, but you mustn't get your hopes up. Now, have you any questions to ask me?'
Mary (getting to her feet): 'No, I don't think so. We must away now and get our bus – I'll ring tonight and again tomorrow. We won't come in tomorrow, we need to sort out things at home.'

We all get up to leave with her. Mary and her daughter leave first.

Consultant C holds the door for us and catches my eye – he frowns and raises his eyebrows and shakes his head, seemingly with discomfort and slight annoyance at her 'matter-of-fact' response.

Mary and her daughter do not return to the hospital until two days later. Again Mary makes it known that they do not wish to stay for too long and this is a cause of anxiety and concern to the intensive care staff. In explaining her desire to leave, Mary describes to me how she believes they should *'keep a grip on normal life, because this isn't normal is it?'* However, S, the nurse caring for John, appears worried when Mary tells her of her intention to leave and suggests that she fetches the registrar to 'fill her in' with regard to John's condition:

S asks them at this point whether they would like to speak to the registrar.

Mary: 'No, we can see how he is – we're going home now and we will be back on Monday. We'll 'phone tomorrow but we won't come in because it's Sunday.'

S looks slightly worried and disappears briefly; she comes back with the registrar. The registrar suggests to Mary that it would be a good idea if he 'fills them in' with how John is. They agree, and he and S disappear with Mary and her daughter. I do not go with them but the registrar and S tell me later that they do not think that Mary 'really grasps how ill he is'.

(From the field notes)

This scene is repeated two days later, on day seven of John's illness. Mary sits beside John's bed and talks brightly to Nurse J, who is looking after him. Her conversation concerns various subjects, but she does not seem to wish to talk about John. Nurse J encourages her to wait and speak to Consultant B about John's condition before she leaves. Mary agrees. I am present during this interview and record my impression that Mary seems almost disinterested in Consultant B's careful account of John's condition. She thanks him for 'all that you are doing', but again gets to her feet to leave when he asks her whether there is anything she would like to ask. Consultant B is concerned by her behaviour and tells Nurse J and myself that he thinks she *'does not really understand what is happening'* and that he *'can't make her out'*.

Mary's apparently unemotional stance when receiving information about her husband and her rejection of attempts to encourage her to stay at his bedside are seen by the staff as puzzling behaviour. They interpret her actions and attitude as a lack of understanding about the seriousness of her husband's condition, and redouble their efforts to facilitate her realization of his probable death. In my subsequent interview with her five months later, Mary's recollections of her experiences in intensive care enable a very different interpretation to be made. She recalls how the environment of intensive care did not *'affect her'* because John had been ill so many times before and therefore she was familiar with the surroundings of intensive care. She then goes on to say that for her, John had died before he reached the Eastern intensive care unit:

> M: I knew when he left X [hospital in hometown] that there wasn't much chance, but to me he more or less died here in X and in the Eastern they were only keeping him alive there artificially. I realized there wouldn't be much chance you know . . . I felt like it had happened here in X and I knew this was going to be the end result. I wish now that I hadn't agreed to, er, taking him to the Eastern and he'd just died here in X. I mean [he] would have loved it, being attached to all that machinery, he loved all that sort of thing you know, but the chances of him pulling through were very small.
>
> JS: And how do you feel about that now?
>
> M: I wish I hadn't gone with him, I wish [children] hadn't seen him in intensive care in the state that he was in because to me he'd died here in X and he was only being kept alive artificially -- I don't think it was very fair in some respects you know, I don't really know.
>
> JS: What was not fair?
>
> M: To keep a person alive like that, when there's not much chance for them at all. As I say I'm sure [my husband] would have been delighted for all the machinery and everything that was going on, you know; but it's not a natural process.
>
> (From follow-up interview)

This extract gives a picture of Mary having to endure the 'unnatural' process of prolonging her husband's life, when to her, he had already died in his home-town hospital. She is concerned about the effect on her children and wishes that he had never been transferred to receive all the 'artificial' treatment, seeing the whole experience as 'unfair'. This information throws a different slant on her apparent lack of understanding and allows a different interpretation to be made. The efforts of the intensive care staff to encourage her to be with John, to sit with him and to listen to explanations about his condition may now be seen as attempts to reproduce the social presence of an individual who, for his wife, has already died. The combined efforts of the intensive care staff to prolong John's life with technology and to facilitate her level of understanding become almost an irrelevance to Mary. As a result she does not react in the way that the staff expect and their attempts to apprehend 'John' through her emotional response to information given about his illness are rendered invalid. She describes, for example, how the information that she was given merely confirmed that which she knew already:

> I was taken into the little interview room and he [one of the doctors] told me then, you know, what I already knew, I mean he was only sort of confirming what was wrong with him, you know, but he was very good. He was trying to explain to me how ill he was but I knew already.
>
> (From follow-up interview)

In this data we begin to see the depth of the complexities involved in the assessment of, and response to, patients' companions by healthcare staff. This is especially the case in situations where only transitory contact takes place. We have seen the potential break in understanding that can emerge during the process of delivering information and support to patients' companions. Further, this data suggests that in some cases efforts that focus on the development of anticipatory grief within companions are misplaced. In this example, Mary *resists* the attempts of the healthcare staff to 'prepare' her for the likelihood of her husband's death. She apprehends their well-meaning efforts to bring her to 'open awareness' of his poor condition as almost an irrelevance, since this episode of acute illness follows years of a disabling, chronic condition during which she had both expected, and prepared for, his death. Further, she has other pressing concerns of a practical and financial nature that seem to overshadow her need for information regarding the severity of John's condition.

Participation in decision making

Up to now, this chapter has explored and deconstructed how staff respond to what they perceive to be the needs of patients' companions for knowledge about prognosis and treatment plans. The complexities involved in this process have been highlighted by the examples of two cases and it has been shown that the relationship between the disclosure of information and the emergence of any ability or desire to influence care decisions is far from straightforward. 'Mismatched' perceptions between healthcare staff and patients' companions regarding the nature and course of the illness have been identified as of particular relevance, together with the problematic process of achieving an appropriate level and style of information disclosure in the face of extreme distress.

Attention now turns to a closer examination of how there is apparently no *overt* attempt on the part of the healthcare staff to encourage companions to influence or control the decision-making process. Insights from earlier studies suggest that what occurs instead is an attempt to remove the 'burden' of decision making, whilst keeping families fully informed about the gravity of the patients' condition. This tendency may be associated with beliefs about the impact of 'guilt' on long-term psychological health and with assumptions about companions' abilities to understand and evaluate complex clinical information (Degner and Beaton 1987). Anspach's (1993) ethnographic study of neonatal intensive care supports this point. Anspach described interactional processes of 'diffusing dissent' and 'producing assent' whereby health professionals maintained control of treatment decisions around critically ill babies: 'staff anticipate, deflect and pre-empt dissent – they attempt to persuade parents to accept their point of view; and when that fails, they neutralize dissent by psychologizing' (Anspach 1993: 130).

Anspach also charts how the delivery of information to parents follows a long process of discussion between health professionals and shows how the unstated aim of healthcare staff and parent meetings is merely to elicit agreement to decisions that have been made already. Rier, in an account of his recollections of his own critical illness, suspects that this technique was adopted during his own illness, and used to make his wife and he *feel* involved in the decision-making process associated with his treatment (2000: 76). In my own study, this strategy was observed most clearly in intensive care in the case of Mr Hart, who had a severe head injury and from whom life-supporting treatment was withdrawn after eight days. Mr Hart was transferred from intensive care and died shortly afterwards on a general ward. Shortly before Mr Hart's transfer to the ward, a series of these exchanges occurs, which results in an agreed plan of treatment withdrawal. During these exchanges, the difficult process of ascertaining that death was inevitable is achieved, in part, by a negotiated dispersal of responsibility between Mr Hart's family and the healthcare staff. In the following extract, a senior consultant, who has not met Mr Hart or his family before, attempts to facilitate a situation whereby agreement is reached between medical, nursing staff and the family to the effect that once Mr Hart's endo-tracheal tube is removed, a tracheostomy *should not* be performed. In this process, the consultant appears to 'allow' Mr Hart's nurse and family to influence the course of events. In this way, the responsibility for the withdrawal of treatments is shared between them all, and it is finally recognized *formally* that death will occur:

Consultant B arrives with the senior registrar and the registrar. The registrar presents Mr Hart's case since she admitted him. Consultant B (there has been a different consultant for each of the days he has been in ITU) takes out the notes and looks at the CT scan films. 'Very severe contusions' he says to the senior registrar who nods and confirms that the neurosurgeons have said this. Consultant B goes to Mr Hart and examines his response to painful stimuli. Mr Hart responds slightly by flexing his legs. When the consultant pulls gently on his endo-tracheal tube he coughs very slightly. Consultant B disconnects

Mr Hart from the ventilator briefly – Mr Hart breathes easily himself. Consultant B moves from the bed and says: 'Right, let's look at his X-rays.' The company moves to the side corridor to the X-ray display board. They briefly look at the X-rays and then Consultant B turns to the registrar and asks: 'What is the definition of a persistent vegetative state?' The registrar answers and they then discuss his age, his prognosis and the fact his Glasgow Coma Score was less than 5 on Accident and Emergency admission.

They discuss the difference between euthanasia and withdrawal of treatment – Consultant B: 'eventually someone will sue us for murder or manslaughter, but the ruling from the Tony Bland case is that medical treatment can be withdrawn if it is in the best interests of the patient. There is no difference in principle between stopping naso-gastric feeding or renal support, and taking someone's e.t. [endo-tracheal] tube out, but many people feel unhappy about the latter because the end comes quickly rather than over the course of several hours.

Consultant to Registrar: 'What do you think we should do?'
Registrar: 'Well I think we could put a tracheostomy in – but then maybe, I'm not sure – perhaps it will just prolong things. We would need to think about what we would do if he develops a chest infection. We need to see what his family thinks.'

Consultant B repeats the question to Staff Nurse Y who replies that: 'His family have been told that he will have a tracheostomy and go to the ward.'

In response to the same question the senior registrar says: 'Well I think that on balance we should not do a tracheostomy but we should wait and see whether he manages alone. What do you think?' (To Consultant B)

Consultant B: 'I think that it is not in his interest to have an extra operation – in a way that is the most comfortable option, but I think it may just prolong the inevitable. That is what I want to speak to the family about.'

(From the field notes)

Consultant B can be seen here clearly directing and drawing together the opinions of the other staff. Both his awareness of, and misgivings about, the current legislative position on the withdrawal of 'extraordinary' treatment allows him to clarify what he sees as the boundaries of permissible action in Mr Hart's case. The senior registrar quickly follows his lead and the registrar also acquiesces, having voiced the opinion that the views of the family should be sought. The consultant then asks Staff Nurse Y about her opinion. It is difficult to detect a personal viewpoint in her response, instead she seems to attempt to represent the knowledge and views of Mrs Hart and Michael.

> *Staff Nurse Y:* '*They have clearly said that they do not want his life to be prolonged if he is not going to recover.*'
>
> (From the field notes)

This mobilization of the views of Mr Hart's wife and son allows Consultant B to outline his favoured plan of action. He leaves to discuss the situation with a consultant colleague. On his return, he tells the staff nurse:

> '*the current situation will be explained to the family, and in 24–36 hours the endo-tracheal tube will be removed to see if he can manage. It will not be replaced, a tracheostomy will not be made and a pneumonia will not be treated.*'
>
> (From the field notes)

In the interview that follows with Mrs Hart and with Michael, Consultant B spends 15–20 minutes explaining in detail the clinical evidence available and the difference between brainstem and cortical function. In the following extract he outlines the options that he has considered and makes his opinion known to Michael and Mrs Hart. They express support for the course of action he recommends and in so doing assume some of the responsibility for the decision to withdraw medical treatment from Mr Hart:

> *[Consultant B talking to Mrs Hart and Michael, outlining the various paths of action/non-action that are possible.]*
>
> '*We could do a small operation called a tracheostomy which would enable him to keep his airway clear and enable him to breathe more easily. We could decide to remove the ET [endo-tracheal] tube. We know that he can breathe because we disconnected him from the ventilator during the ward round today – and see how he gets on. If we took this course then we would let nature take its course. We would not replace the tube and we would not treat any pneumonia that may develop. Option 1 is perhaps the easiest option, but it would probably just prolong the inevitable. Option 2 would mean that he might only manage for a couple of hours, but this is uncertain; he might be able to manage for a long period of time. It is our opinion, and I have discussed this with Dr X, that option 2 is the best course of action.*'
>
> *Mrs Hart and Michael:* '*Oh yes, please, please, do that – we have been through all this together and we don't want him to be left like he is: he wouldn't have wanted that.*'
>
> (From the field notes)

Michael's retrospective account of events, given in an interview four months after his father's death, suggests that he valued the opportunity to assume some of the responsibility for the course of action taken. He felt that he and his mother were given the opportunity to veto the consultant's plan:

> I dare say, in fact I know it, if we had insisted and gone along the lines there is no way we are giving in, he would still have been alive on a machine now -- but, as you know yourself, the way we talked about it, *we* thought it was better for the person, my dad, to let him go because he wouldn't have wanted to be in the state, what do you call -- ? Persistent vegetative state or anything like it.
>
> (From follow-up interview)

In her follow-up interview, Mrs Hart is similarly clear about her willingness to take part in the decision-making process. Indeed she seems to recall playing a central role in that process and relates this to fulfilling her responsibilities towards her husband:

> When the doctor said there wasn't much hope and they didn't think he was going to make it, the decision was mine, whether to carry on with the treatment or to let it go and I thought, well, would (he) want to lay there for evermore being turned and handled, being no good . . . it was a big decision to make, but it was the only thing to do. (For him), no matter how it hurt me, it was the right thing to do, for him you know.
>
> (From follow-up interview)

It can therefore be seen how in some cases clinicians are able to diffuse responsibility for death by drawing nurses and patients' families into the decision-making process. Where the recognition of 'dying' occurs at a relatively early point and is shared by all parties, it seems that conditions are created for the successful apportioning of responsibility between the healthcare staff and families. However, it must be noted that the unfolding course of events is not altered in any fundamental way by this redistribution of responsibility. In some situations, in spite of a general strategy of eliciting agreement to decisions that have been made already, companions are able to alter critically the course of decisions taken around the ill person. Anspach (1993) observed how parents' influence was 'allowed' when there was a degree of uncertainty over the correctness of a particular decision, and in those circumstances when the parents were perceived as particularly 'competent' to participate: perhaps by virtue of some specialized medical knowledge. In my own study, I observed similarly that 'critical moments' can arise in which families take the opportunity to intervene. Staff then follow their lead in carrying out a plan of action more decisively than might otherwise have been the case. Enormous courage is required on the part of families taking this type of action.

Influencing non-treatment decisions: Mrs Taylor's case

We now rejoin the activities around Mrs Taylor. It was noted in Chapter 3 that the intensive care staff had come to an agreement that intensive care was no longer appropriate or meaningful in Mrs Taylor's case. The consultant asked the senior registrar to make arrangements to transfer her to a ward so that 'nature can take its course'.

Mrs Taylor's management was marked by the characteristic style of 'pessimistic' communication, which involved the intensive care staff placing a repeated emphasis on the gravity of her condition and on the limits of possible medical treatment. Both concern and embarrassment were expressed by the nursing and medical staff when Mrs Taylor's husband engaged with what they perceived to be inappropriately optimistic beliefs concerning his wife's illness and when this occurred their efforts to ensure that he understood the 'reality' of the situation were re-doubled. To this effect the nursing staff encouraged him to visit and sit with his wife, and they organized consultations with the medical staff to ensure that he received information about his wife's prognosis. Eventually these efforts, in my interpretation, seemed to engender the conditions in which Mr Taylor and his family suggested for themselves that further treatments (namely the tracheostomy procedure) should not be carried out. This critical intervention had the ultimate effect of dispersing the responsibility for the withholding of treatment from Mrs Taylor between the intensive care staff and her family. It led to a final limiting of medical treatment and was characterized as 'surprising' by the senior registrar involved and as 'brave' by the nurse on duty that day.

Mr Taylor seemed ill at ease with the communicative efforts of the healthcare staff and at a loss to know how to behave towards his wife in such an alien environment. For example, the following extract is taken from the field notes on day 16, a few hours after Mrs Taylor had been extubated:

17:00 – Mr Taylor has come to visit. He sits holding his wife's hand: he has to lean across the cot sides to do this. He tries to speak to and smile at her. She responds weakly. He doesn't seem to know what to do and lapses into what seems uncomfortable silence. He sits with his head down, but maintains his grip on her hand. The SR goes and speaks to him; he listens while she explains how she is and that they will have to see how she copes with her breathing.

I speak to him and say hello, he says; 'Well, they've got rid of the tubes but she still doesn't look too good, she doesn't look good to me.' (Mrs Taylor indeed to my eyes looks very tired – she is leaning heavily to the left and breathing noisily with her mouth wide open under the mask – she looks at him but does not hold his gaze when he speaks to her.)

Mr Taylor leaves after three quarters of an hour. He kisses her, squeezes her hands and speaks to her encouragingly. Then he leaves quickly without looking behind him.

(From the field notes)

The anxiety of the healthcare staff to communicate the 'realities' of Mrs Taylor's illness to her husband appeared to be related to their concern to facilitate his assent to what they saw as the most likely outcome: a decision to withdraw or withhold treatments from Mrs Taylor. They entreated Mr Taylor to engage in repeated conversations and tried to get him to stay at his wife's bedside. However, in my interpretation, he appeared confused by their repeated emphases on the severity of her illness on the one hand and the delivery of highly technological, active treatments on the other. Such inconsistency seemed to overwhelm him, and he appeared powerless to make his own opinions known. He fell back instead on ideas from astrology, referring to the influence of the 'new moon' on his wife's chances of recovery. Such 'magic' was, for him, in the same category of explanation as the health technology he witnessed being used on his wife. His body language, however, belied any faith he may have had in either health technology or astrology as a potential saviour. His discomfiture, his agitated attempts to comfort his wife and his rapid departure without a backward glance seemed, in my interpretation, to be the actions of someone trying to say a final goodbye. This was an impression also gained by Mrs Taylor's primary nurse. Shortly after my observation of his sad departure, she speaks to me about her belief that Mrs Taylor's treatment is too subjective (see Chapter 3), and she tells me that she believes that Mr Taylor is: *'just tolerating all of this – I'd like to know what's going on in his head'* (field note, day 17).

As outlined in Chapter 3, Mrs Taylor's condition gradually deteriorates and it is decided during a ward round to perform a mini-tracheostomy on her before transferring her to a ward. The senior registrar is asked by the duty consultant to prepare for this by speaking to Mr Taylor and to the surgeons (to whose ward she will be transferred). Mr Taylor has arrived to visit, this time with his brother and sister-in-law. The following is an extract from the field notes taken on that day describing the interview between Mr Taylor and the senior registrar:

Having asked the permission of the SR to be present at the interview with Mr Taylor if he agrees, I then continue helping to prepare bed 4. I am able to see Mr Taylor and his sister-in-law come in and sit down next to Mrs Taylor. They speak to her but she makes no response. Mr Taylor sits closest to the head of the bed and sits with his hands in his lap and his head down. His sister-in-law looks upset and repeatedly strokes and squeezes Mrs Taylor's hand.

The SR calls to me quietly: 'I'm going to speak to them now. Where's Nurse C?'

(Nurse C is behind the curtains helping with the new patient.) She comes out and tells Mr Taylor that the doctor would like to speak to them. I take my chance and ask Mr Taylor if I may accompany them, he says: 'Yes, of course.'

As we move to the interview room Mr Taylor speaks to another older man: 'Come on, you come too.' He tells us: 'This is my brother.'

We all go to the interview room, and everyone sits down.

The SR begins by saying: 'Well, I expect you've noticed that she is not so well today; we're not sure why that is. It could be that she has had another stroke, or it could be that the infection in her tummy is returning. You do know, I think, that we have not managed to clear her pneumonia completely?'

Mr Taylor: 'Yes, yes, I know that'. (His relatives nod)

SR: 'Well, our plan is to do a mini-trache -- (she stops, realizing that they will not understand this term and starts again) -- to make a little hole in her windpipe so that we can clear her secretions . . . and then, I think we will transfer her from here to a surgical ward. I don't think ITU is the place for her now.'

Mr Taylor: 'Well, you know best don't you?' (he says this gruffly, as if struggling to maintain his composure)

There follows a short, but strained silence, as if he is trying to say something, eventually his sister-in-law, who has been looking at him, speaks: 'It seems a shame really to keep on doing things to her – she wouldn't want it would she?'

Mr Taylor (shaking his head): 'No, she wouldn't.'

SR: 'So how do you feel about that?'

There is a pause again, and then the sister-in-law speaks again: 'Well, I don't think she's going to get any better now is she?'

Brother: 'See -- she's got so many things wrong with her: just one and she might have had a chance; but I know that [Mr Taylor] has been so worn down by the strain of caring for her: she's had two strokes and really didn't go out at all at home.'

Sister-in-law: 'People were always asking how she was – never how Mr Taylor was, and yet it's the carers that take all the strain. He used to cry because of it.'

Mr Taylor is silent, but is looking increasingly upset.

SR: 'Well, I think I gather from what you are saying to me that you feel that we shouldn't do the tracheostomy – it is quite an invasive thing to do.'

Mr Taylor speaks at last: 'She looks comfortable today, let's just let her go, drift away now.'
Sister and brother: 'Yes, that's right, as long as she doesn't suffer.'
SR: 'Well, I will have to speak to my consultant and we will discuss this. Of course, she may pull round from this, but I doubt it. I think from our discussion today we should just see how things go?'
Mr Taylor: 'Yes, that's right.'

(From field notes, day 17)

Here the senior registrar's presentation to Mr Taylor and his brother and sister-in-law seems tentative and slightly nervous, as if she expects them to disagree with the plan to transfer Mrs Taylor from intensive care. In my interpretation, her careful explanation about Mrs Taylor's continuing pneumonia and identification of her other clinical problems seems to be an attempt to encourage the family to accept the plan agreed on the ward round and to avert the possibility of any conflict due to the family's wish to increase or re-institute the intensive care therapies being given to Mrs Taylor. The unexpected intervention of the sister-in-law and the gruff response of Mr Taylor: *'You know best don't you?'* tells a different story however. Taking these actions with the earlier observations in which Mr Taylor appeared to prepare for his wife's death and eventually bid a final goodbye to her; it appears that the response to the senior registrar was a planned attempt (that took considerable courage) to ensure that Mrs Taylor was allowed to die without further medical interventions. In her follow-up interview the senior registrar recalled how surprised she was with the reaction of the Taylors:

I mean, I had always, up until that point, assumed that they were relatives who were very, very, keen that everything be done until the very last moment; and I think in my mind I had already got to the point of thinking, 'we're not really winning here'; but I thought the relatives were going to be pushing and pushing for the absolute maximum to be done and my worry at that point was that they were going to want her to be put back onto the ventilator if the new tracheostomy didn't work. So, I was actually waiting for them to come back at me with: 'What's going to happen if this mini-trache doesn't work?', which is the ground I was testing. I was completely taken by surprise by finding in fact that they had actually reached their own point of being ready to, to not continue with aggressive treatment . . . all the way through her husband had been told that her chances were poor and yet he seemed to be (pause) in a different world and so I assumed that he had continued to have that hopefulness of her recovery.

(From follow-up interview)

Here the senior registrar confirms that the intention in warning Mr Taylor of his wife's poor 'chances' had been to prepare the way for any expression of dissent from him, and that during this interview she was still 'testing the ground' to see if the expected conflict would materialize. It is ironic, then, that it was at this point that he and his family interrupted the gradual movement towards a full cessation of medical treatments being orchestrated by the healthcare staff and precipitated an earlier withdrawal of treatment from Mrs Taylor than would have occurred otherwise. Their intervention was met with relief by the healthcare staff. Staff Nurse C, for example, remarked afterwards: 'I thought they were really brave, I thought for a minute that they weren't going to say anything.' Such relief seemed to indicate the willing acceptance by the healthcare staff of shared moral responsibility between themselves and the family for the final withdrawal of treatments that then occurred.

Discussion

The management of clinical decisions about the withdrawal or withholding of treatment such that hopelessly ill people can die 'naturally' remains extremely complex. Enduring diagnostic difficulties can make it difficult to predict accurately that someone is 'dying', and thus affect the degree to which clinicians can begin to shift their emphasis to palliative, rather than curative care. Further, the diagnosis of dying may often only be made by exclusion (Blackburn 1989), leaving little time for the careful and compassionate communications between patient, family and healthcare staff on which good 'person-centred' clinical care depends. Among patients admitted to intensive care, diagnostic difficulty is compounded by the constraints of complex life-support therapies, the prognostic consequences of which are difficult to apprehend. These not only render patient–clinician communication almost impossible, but also complicate the whole process of 'sharing knowledge' and developing a mutual understanding. Moreover, the speed with which patients' conditions change in intensive care can force the pace and demand a more paternalistic and apparently controlling clinical response than that which may be possible in environments where clinical changes occur more slowly.

Conjoined with these issues are those of the vulnerability engendered by sudden immersion in an alien environment and the ordeal of witnessing the dying and death of a close companion. Indeed, the variable tension between the feeling of 'vulnerability' and the desire to take 'control' (Lupton 1996) has been little examined, but may be an important contributor to the very individual response produced by the prospect of death and the experience of critical illness (Rier 2000). It may also explain why, in this study, some companions welcomed the way in which 'treatment options' were outlined by certain consultants because this gave them a sense of involvement and they seemed later (in their follow-up interviews) to be able to assert a belief that they had been given the chance to act in what they perceived to be their relatives' best interest. This was perceived as a final exercise of familial responsibility and love for the dying person. Other respondents, in contrast, seemed to welcome, and be comforted by, the very firm guidance and control of the medical staff.

It can be argued on the basis of these observations that care decisions must take account of companions' need for expert guidance, but in a manner in which their position as 'next of kin' is fully acknowledged. Nelson and Nelson (1995) have suggested a wholesale re-examination of the role of the patient's next of kin in care decision making. In this, they argue, the accepted paternalistic position of medicine and its role in 'presenting' the patient's best interests to companions/families would be replaced and subjected to critical scrutiny. Instead of presentation, an in-depth exploration of understanding would be undertaken. This would allow not only for the production of a 'shared narrative' and understanding (Karlawish 1996) of illness, but also for a more equitable contribution to end-of-life decisions. Such a process would not lead to a dereliction of duty for the physician, but would facilitate a trusting relationship and a more individual response to the particular familial and social circumstances with which illness is surrounded. Such exploration of understanding would facilitate a more 'tailored' response to the experience of loss and grief where the focus would be on responding to the *particular* concerns and feelings of patients' companions.

In this chapter I have discussed the 'front stage' world of intensive care as experienced from the point of view of patients' close companions. Running alongside this world, however, as we have already seen in earlier chapters, is the behind the scenes activity whereby clinicians struggle to establish whether or not death is imminent and try to construct a case that justifies the withdrawal of 'active' medical treatment such that 'natural death' can occur. This is the vexed question of distinguishing between 'killing' and 'letting die' and it is to this that attention now turns.

Note

1 The use of data taken from telephone conversations may be criticized as unethical; however, the intensive care context meant that such calls were in the 'public arena': they were conducted at the central desk and could be heard by everyone on the unit. Further, I decided that in this particular case, the inclusion of the call was important both for clarifying the fragile nature of relationships between staff and companions and in emphasizing the role of telephone conversations in those relationships.

Withdrawing medical treatment
in intensive care: the
problem of 'natural death'

Recent empirical evidence of barriers to palliative care in acute hospital settings shows that dying patients may receive invasive and inappropriate medical treatments in the days and hours before death, in spite of evidence of their poor prognosis being available to clinicians (Faber-Langendoen and Bartels 1992; Principal Investigators for the SUPPORT Project 1995; Ahronheim *et al.* 1996; Faber-Langendoen 1996). The difficulties of ascertaining treatment preferences, predicting the trajectory of dying in critically ill people with complex disease pathologies, and assessing the degree to which further interventions are futile are well documented (Cook 1997; Danis 1998). Further, enduring ethical complexities attending end-of-life care mean that the process of withdrawing or withholding medical treatments is associated with significant problems and risks for clinical staff. Specific difficulties attend the legitimation of treatment withdrawal, the perceived differences between 'killing' and 'letting die' and the cultural constraints that attend the orchestration of 'good' and 'natural' death in situations where human agency is often required before death can follow dying.

This chapter explores the processes by which imminent death is acknowledged by medical staff and decisions are made to withdraw 'active' medical treatment such that 'natural death' can occur. In the discussion of the construction of prognostic certainty (Chapter 3), it was suggested that medical knowledge about individuals is a negotiated 'product' (Atkinson 1995) in which the meaning of clinical data is open to various interpretations. The focus here is on a closer examination of negotiation within the context of end-of-life decision making in intensive care. The discussion has been informed by the case studies of eight patients from whom treatment was withdrawn shortly before death, although again 'critical cases' are used to explore themes of more general applicability. Analysis of data relating to this issue was informed by an extensive literature review of the 'problem' of non-treatment decisions in intensive care, and other 'acute' areas of hospital care. A résumé of these sources follows.

Non-treatment decisions in intensive care: insights from the literature

Patients admitted to intensive care comprise critically ill individuals with a complex mix of acute and chronic pathologies. Of these, between 15 and 35 per cent die during intensive therapy (Koch *et al.* 1994; Metcalfe and McPherson 1994; Gunning and Rowan 1999), and formal medical decisions to limit or withdraw treatments habitually precede death (Smedira *et al.* 1990; Koch *et al.* 1994; Simpson 1994; Searle 1996; Winter and Cohen 1999). This mirrors a trend visible in the management of death within other hospital areas (Faber-Langendoen and Bartels 1992; Pijnenborg *et al.* 1995; Faber-Langendoen 1996). In spite of their increasing incidence, little is known about the processes of withdrawing or withholding medical treatment. Winter and Cohen suggest, however, that 'the timing of withdrawal, the treatments withdrawn, and the manner of withdrawal may vary considerably, not only from country to country but also between intensive care units in the same country' (1999: 306).

One reason for variation between countries comes from differences in the law surrounding end-of-life decision making. A major difference between the UK and the US, for example, rests on the concept of surrogacy for patients who are too ill to be able to make informed autonomous decisions about their own treatment. In some American states, a designated chain of surrogacy exists and it is a legal obligation of clinicians to consult with the designated surrogate before making any treatment decision. In the UK, close companions and relatives have no legal right of surrogacy, although recent guidance on end-of-life decision making from the British Medical Association (1999) probably reflects current practice in its advice that they have a pivotal role to play in informing the deliberations of clinicians about patients' best interests, capacity to benefit and quality of life. The previous chapter highlighted the relationship between close companions and clinicians, and examined some of the difficulties that may arise.

Some evidence is available which suggests that differences in processes of decision making between intensive care units in the same country may be due to organizational and cultural norms that develop. These influence the manner in which non-treatment decisions are approached and enacted. Thus, in a comparative study of two intensive care units in the US, Zussman (1992) demonstrates that the physicians in one unit not only made non-treatment decisions more frequently, but also followed a more decisive style in implementing those decisions. Zussman draws on the early work of

Sudnow, who observed how staff interact on the basis that 'death must be made to seem an outcome of dying' (1967: 95), and describes how some 30 years later:

> In the face of uncertainty, physicians struggle to maintain discretion. They do so, in part, by conceptualizing both the course of the illness and the types of treatment in terms that allow wide latitude in judgements as to what constitutes 'appropriate' action. This strategy is evident in the ways physicians conceptualize 'terminal'. It is also evident in the distinction they make between 'aggressive' and 'unaggressive' treatments.
>
> (Zussman 1992: 123)

In a comparative ethnography of intensive care and obstetric settings in the UK, Harvey (1997) sheds further light on the variation in action and approach to non-treatment decisions, describing how clinical staff in intensive care engage in a strategic practice of withdrawing life support slowly in order to mimic the decline of 'natural' death and in accordance with culturally prescriptive norms about the proper course of 'natural' dying. Similarly, Slomka (1992) describes the 'bargaining' or 'negotiation' process that occurs at the bedside of a critically ill person. Such bargaining defines the meaning of medical technology, and helps to decide 'how far medical technology should go in prolonging life or in prolonging death' (1992: 251). Slomka points to the way in which moral responsibility for the patient's death by withdrawing treatment is shared with family members, while the moral responsibility for the patient's death by withholding treatment is displaced to the patient.

In a study of the use of resuscitation procedures and equipment in the construction of 'dignified death' in the emergency room, Timmermans (1998) notes the complex intersection between human agency and technological power in Western secularized cultures, in which resuscitation techniques have become incorporated into a dense pattern of cultural beliefs about death with dignity. In this patterning of beliefs, rather than technology being inimical to dignified death, it takes a central role in the procurement of dignity in the event of sudden, traumatic deaths and is used to make sense of deaths that might otherwise seem meaningless. This can lead to variation in practice according to the particular circumstances in which death occurs, and according to the motivations and understandings of those involved in resuscitative attempts.

Against the backdrop of culturally and morally prescriptive ideas about 'natural' death, the role of technology in this event and the part played by different actors, extensive concerns have been expressed by clinicians regarding the legal and ethical implications of such issues. Most frequently expressed is a concern over the philosophical 'shades of grey' that surround the distinction between euthanasia and withdrawal of treatment. This has been described as the distinction between 'killing and letting die' (Rachels 1975; Johnson 1993; McMahon 1993; Cartwright 1996). The uncertainty surrounding the distinction has led to attempts to ensure that there is no 'proximate relationship' (Hoyt 1995: 621), or apparently causative link, between the withdrawal of life support and death. A central aspect of this discussion is the difficulty of predicting whether or not a particular course of action is prolonging inevitable death or facilitating all the chances for 'meaningful' recovery.

In an early commentary, Jennett framed the essential dilemma in intensive care as 'the vicious circle of commitment' (1984: 1709), pointing out that the withdrawal of therapy, *even when* it is agreed that the prognosis is 'hopeless', is very much more difficult than taking the decision not even to start such treatment. These complexities are conjoined with a developing awareness among the medical profession that their decisions about the treatment of individual patients or groups of patients may be the subject of challenges from various sources. Such challenges may at times be paradoxical. Thus demands for freedom from medical intervention, perhaps expressed as desires for 'living wills' or 'advance directives', may at the same time be paralleled by demands that doctors preserve life indefinitely. The concept of 'futility' has been employed to describe a scenario in which pressure is exerted on physicians to continue treatment by the companions of fatally ill individuals (Schniederman *et al.* 1990; Teres 1993; Hoyt 1995).

One response to the complex management of non-treatment decisions has been to analyse and discuss the ethical principles on which modern medical practice is based and apply these to the discussion of life and death issues in intensive care (Task Force on Ethics of the Society of Critical Care Medicine 1990). This approach, together with the legal precedents that have emerged from celebrated cases has led to the development of guidelines for use in practical situations. Such guidelines are relatively common in the US, and reflect a growing move towards surrogate decision making in that country (Wanzer *et al.* 1984; Nelson and Nelson 1995). In the UK, guidelines have emerged following the 'increasingly fine line' (P. Bennett 1995), identified in cases such as *Airedale NHS Trust* v *Bland* (1993), between extraordinary and ordinary treatment. For example, following this particular case a 'Practice Note' was issued by the Official Solicitor, which outlines general principles of law as applied to the withdrawal of all forms of treatment from individuals who are diagnosed as being in a persistent vegetative state. Most recently, the British Medical Association has published advice about the withdrawal and withholding of treatment (BMA 1999). However, the extensive legal documentation that surrounds end-of-life decisions in the US is largely absent in the UK. Bayliss identified this difference as early as 1982, and related it to a variety of cultural and social factors. Of these, he identified the developing culture of 'distrust' of medicine in the US as a central contributor to public 'litigiousness' (1982: 1374).

The emergent culture of 'risk' and the extensive attempts to clarify the legal and ethical issues surrounding non-treatment decisions may be related to attempts to develop what some commentators call 'the science of prognosis' (Searle 1996: 291). Such attempts involve the subjugation of the 'art' of medical decision making concerning individual patients to 'scientific guidelines'. The growth of evidence-based medicine is one pre-eminent example of this contemporary preoccupation. Gordon gives a comprehensive review of this trend in medicine, and describes how the 'personal power and private magic' (1988: 257) invested in the clinical judgement of the individual physician has come under attack, with physicians being asked to 'make themselves and their practice more visible' (1988: 257). This involves the application of theories of decision analysis, of epidemiology and of probability, to clinical judgement about individual patients. In intensive care, the trend towards developing severity of illness scores as a predictive tool is a specific illustration of this more general theme (Gunning and Rowan 1999), as are attempts to eradicate the 'prognostic disagreement and inaccuracy' (Poses *et al.* 1989: 827) caused by the idiosyncratic values, beliefs and habits of individual physicians (Poses *et al.* 1989; Christakis and Asch 1993). Gordon also points out that such attempts to 'rationalize' clinical judgement do not sit easily with theories about 'how we know' (1988: 268). These theories emphasize the 'Gestalt' nature of clinical knowledge, which enables the experienced 'expert' to 'zero in' on the meaning of a particular constellation of clinical signs (1988: 276). Gordon describes the 'embodied', phenomenological form of this knowledge and how it is 'sensed through and with the body. This includes senses of sight, sound, touch, smell, as well as emotions and more general senses, such as "feeling that something makes sense", "having a gut feeling" or a sense of salience' (Gordon 1988: 269).

We now turn to focus on the conduct of medical decision making at the bedside of critically ill people, seeing how medical work with dying people in intensive care may be regarded as an interactional accomplishment, which achieves balance between disparate tensions and constraints. The analysis highlights the existence of two potentially divergent dying trajectories: 'technical' and 'bodily'. It appears that these must be aligned in order for death to occur at the 'right' time. Containing and preventing divergence between bodily and technical dying are represented as the basis of 'nature taking its course' and 'natural death' in intensive care. However, the data suggest that 'natural death' is primarily constructed during medical work by means of four interactional strategies, which centre around timing, causation and responsibility.[1] First, the establishment of a 'technical' definition of dying – based on blood results, monitoring evidence and investigation – over and above 'bodily' dying, based on the habitual recognition of the senses and informed by clinical experience. Such definition occurs across a variable time period and involves the active negotiation and re-negotiation of the meaning of medical-technical data. Second, the trajectory of 'known' technical dying is aligned with the development of 'seen' and 'felt' bodily dying to ensure that the events of treatment withdrawal are seen to have no *directly* causative link to death. Third, the problem of causation is further dealt with by a strategic balancing of medical action with medical non-action. This allows for a diffusion of responsibility for death to the body of the ill person, with the body defined as no longer able to take advantage of medical technology. Fourth, medical work is directed, where circumstances allow, towards the incorporation of patients' companions and nursing staff into the decision-making process. These strategies, which enable clinicians to draw dying and death into the 'production' (Atkinson 1995) of 'rational science' and at the same time respond to a complex range of ethical issues *and* cultural beliefs concerning death, were visible in varying degrees of emphasis in all of the eight cases observed in which death followed a non-treatment decision. The last chapter looked at how companions are 'drawn' into the process of decision making, this chapter concentrates on examining the first three strategies outlined above.

Defining 'dying': accomplishing medical work

Material is drawn from three case studies to illuminate the intricacies of medical decision making as it occurs. The extract from the first of these has been chosen since it illustrates how the definition of dying hinges on achieving agreement about the meaning of medical treatment and of medical-technical data. As shown in this case, such agreement *evolves* across time: several days elapsed in this particular example before agreement was reached. It illustrates how 'intuitive' accounts of 'bodily dying' are subsumed to the 'scientific' analysis of 'technical dying'. The second case study extract is similarly illustrative of a negotiated definition of dying, but focuses more closely on the way in which medical action is balanced with non-action such that 'natural death' occurs. In both of the examples the problems of definition are clearly shown between 'withholding', 'withdrawal' and 'euthanasia'.

Negotiating the alignment of bodily and technical dying: John's case

John was admitted to intensive care for treatment for gastro-intestinal bleeding, liver and lung disease. We encountered one aspect of John's management in Chapter 5, in the discussion about the interrelationship between his wife, Mary, and the intensive care staff.

John developed cardiac failure shortly after his admission. During his nine days in intensive care attempts were made to establish a cause for his intestinal bleeding and to treat his developing lung and cardiac failure.

John received ventilation and drainage of a pleural effusion, together with cardiac monitoring and drug support. A gastroscopy was performed soon after his admission to assess his gastro-intestinal bleeding, and he received multiple transfusions of blood and clotting factors. Due to the gravity of his overall condition, he was deemed unsuitable for surgery within the first two days of his treatment following a diagnosis of adult respiratory distress syndrome; continuous veno-venous haemofiltration (similar to dialysis and known as 'CVVH') was commenced on day three. This was used in an attempt to reduce the severe pulmonary oedema and heart failure from which John was suffering as a result of the disease process in his lungs. The CVVH had to be discontinued when his cardiovascular state deteriorated rapidly. John was nursed in a prone position for periods in an attempt to maximize his lung expansion and oxygen exchange but was transferred to a kinetic bed (an automatically tilting bed) because of difficulties in observing him for bleeding in that position. Sedative and paralyzing agents were administered at all times to enable John to tolerate these treatments. When his cardiac and respiratory condition continued to deteriorate, decisions were taken that he was not for resuscitation, for re-institution of CVVH, or for more complex ventilatory procedures. These decisions were taken on day six. Following further intestinal bleeding and development of an intractable cardiac arrhythmia over the course of days eight and nine, cardiac drug support was withdrawn from John. He died during the afternoon of day nine. We join the case on day four.

The following extract comes from the field notes which were taken on that day after the ward round. The notes illustrate how the medical staff consult and negotiate with one another in trying to establish a course of action. Sometimes the consultation is part of the education of junior medical staff, but it also enables the 'smoothing out' of differences of opinion between doctors of equal status, or of different specialties, as to the likely response to a particular therapeutic option. The extract below can be seen as an *active construction* of the nature of John's illness, in which negotiation over the meaning of medical-technical data and of the technical treatments given to John run parallel to, and have to be aligned with, the less easily articulated but clear recognition of inevitable bodily dying. Most noteworthy is the discussion between two consultant anaesthetists, Consultants 'B' and 'C', who struggle to establish a course of action that is scientifically valid but also in keeping with their 'intuitive' recognition of inevitable death. The discussion between them concerns whether John is suffering from multiple 'three-system' organ failure (recognized as a crucial indicator of the statistical probability of death), and the extent to which the CVVH is alleviating or aggravating his heart and respiratory failure. The consultants argue for 15 minutes, trying to interpret highly technical data and agree on a course of therapeutic action, before asking another doctor to settle the disagreement:

14:15 – Consultant C's ward round.

John's family have gone out. Nurse R presents the case. Consultant C listens and looks very grave and concerned. 'This is a very complicated case, what do you think we should do?' (This is directed to the senior registrar and the registrar.) The senior registrar hesitates, the registrar doesn't answer, but she laughs nervously. Consultant C in response to this says: 'No, you can't consider withdrawing, he only has two-system failure – heart and lungs – so what do we do? Are you waiting for me to say?' They assent to this by nodding. Consultant C: 'Well, I think we should stop the CVVH and give him a big bolus of fluid. He has a tachycardia, a low bp [blood pressure] and a low wedge [indirect measurement of left heart pressure] which has not responded to adrenaline or dobutamine. Give him 500 mls of hespan and 500 mls of HAS [both colloid solutions] and we will retrack [measure physiological data] him at 16:00.'

Nurse R: 'Shall we stop the CVVH now?'

Consultant C: 'Wait for a bit – I think it should come off, but I need to discuss it with Consultant B' (who is not there, and who had been adamant that the CVVH should remain – I wonder whether this accounts for the nervousness of the registrar and the senior registrar.)

14:45 – The surgical senior registrar and lecturer appear. They sit and read John's file and then go behind the curtains to examine him. They question Nurse R as to his condition. Just then Consultant C comes out of the side-room, sees them and comes across to speak to them. There is some discussion about his liver function and the presence or not of varices: 'I didn't see any on scope' and: 'I don't believe all of this written in the notes' and 'Has he had a splenectomy or not?' There is much rustling of paper, trying to make sense of previous notes. The surgeon then says that in his opinion there is still no possibility of surgical intervention at the moment because of his poor state and that it is not clear that he needs surgery anyway, since they still do not really know what is wrong with him. Consultant B appears at the end of this discussion and listens. The surgeons then leave and Consultants C and B are left together.

Consultant C says to Consultant B: 'I think he is intravascularly dry, so I am loading him with fluid – it's had an effect already, and I'd like to take him off of the CVVH now.'

Consultant B – looking unhappy and very concerned – 'The problem is that the colloid doesn't stay where we want it to for long, it moves into the interstitial space and then we are back to where we started. I think we need to fill him, but take off fluid at the same time.'

Consultant C: 'I agree with you, but I feel that he crashes [becomes severely hypoxic and hypotensive] on being put onto CVVH – it's too aggressive. He is peeing – we should rely on that. Dr X always says, if one thing doesn't work try something else and if that works, pursue it. I mean each patient is different, they do not respond in a predictable, linear way to intervention.'

Consultant B: 'Yes, I can't disagree with you – it's just that, well, I just feel, we should keep the CVVH going, theoretically it should work.'

Consultant C: 'What we are debating is the whole crux of ITU medicine – intravascular v interstitial fluid movement. Basically, no one knows what it is best to do.'

Consultant B: (turns to the senior registrar who has been listening while taking blood and collecting data for the 'tracking'): 'What do you think Dr . . . ?'

Senior Registrar: 'Well, he's very poorly.' (smiling)

Hoots of laughter all round.

The senior registrar becomes more serious: '. . . but I think he has responded to fluid and we should take the CVVH off.'

Consultant C (lowering his voice): 'Look, we all know that this man is going to die – he has all the hallmarks, we all know the ones who don't make it – but he only has two-system failure, lungs and heart, so we've got to carry on trying – I don't think it will do any good.'

Consultant B: 'I agree with you, I think he will die, but we've got to carry on trying.'

(From the field notes, day 4)

The use of humour in this example has the effect of undermining the extensive technical debate and legitimating 'intuitive' beliefs that John will almost certainly die. It allows the consultants to express to each other their private recognition of the likelihood, indeed the certainty, of John's bodily dying. However, in spite of this sudden expression of resistance to medical-technical discourse, they are unable to justify action on the basis of 'seen' bodily dying. Full treatment is continued.

John's condition stabilizes briefly over the course of day five, but he suffers a further episode of acute deterioration during the early hours of day six. The consultants featured in the earlier exchange are now off duty and the management of John's care has been delegated to the on-call consultant, senior registrar, and the registrar. The following extract from the field notes demonstrates the way these individuals achieve a re-definition of John's clinical data, which enables them to justify decisions to *withhold* particular types of treatment from him:

Senior Registrar: 'I just feel that we're going nowhere. He is on maximal support, and I just think he is going to die. I believe that he

*would have a less than 10 per cent chance of survival if he only had
a lung injury of the type he has, without all of the other problems.'*
Registrar: *'The problem is Consultant B; he does not want us to withdraw on this man. He says that as there is only two-system failure
we should continue treatment – look it's written here.' All three read
the 'file' [medical notes].*
Senior Registrar: *'Well, I think he has liver failure as well.'*
Registrar: *'That hasn't been such a problem apparently.'*
Consultant: *'Let's have a look.' (He turns to the biochemistry and
haematology results flow sheet.)*
Senior Registrar: *'Look! How can it be said that he is not in liver failure
with figures like that! (He points to the bilirubin and plasma protein
results.)*
Consultant: *'OK, we all know that this man is going to die, but it
depends on how far you want to push it. You could argue the toss
with Consultant B, or you can decide not to do certain things. Are
you going to CVVH him if he develops renal failure for example?'*
Senior Registrar: *'No.'*
Consultant: *'Right, OK, are you going to jet him?' [This unusual 'last
chance' form of artificial ventilation was discussed earlier as a possible option.]*
Senior Registrar: *'There is no point because his prognosis is so appalling.'*
Consultant: *'Right, he is on maximal support already then. I don't
think it's a question of withdrawing that. Will you resuscitate him if
he arrests?'*
Senior Registrar: *'There won't be any point, he won't recover.'*
Consultant: *'So, he's not for resuscitation. There is nothing more that
you can do.'*

(From the field notes, day 6)

This ward round has the effect of extending the limits of medical action
from surgical intervention to the more fundamental technique of resuscitation. This limitation hinges on the diagnosis of liver failure, which removes
John from the realms of the potentially salvageable 'two-system' failure
category, into the potentially unsalvageable 'three-system' failure category.
The manner in which haematological and biochemical data are debated
reveals clearly that such figures are open to various interpretations according to the standpoint of the individual reading them. In this way, the intuitive knowledge based on past clinical experience – *'we all know this man is
going to die'* – is gradually aligned to the demonstrable technical and biomedical data, and the conditions that allow them to devise a plan of *non-
action* are established. The medical support he is already receiving becomes
defined as 'maximal' and the duty consultant is able to reassure the senior
registrar and registrar that *'there is nothing more you can do'*.

The following day (day seven, when Consultant B is back on duty) there are further discussions relating to the haematological and biochemical data, again indicating the variability of interpretations that are possible on the basis of such data, and the differential evaluations that can be made when such figures are 'read' alongside the results from other diagnostic investigations. At this point, Consultant B persists in his opinion that John's liver function is 'holding its own', and instead concentrates on the severity of his lung disease as demonstrated by the series of chest X-rays available. This difference in opinion means that while the plan for *non-action* outlined above is adhered to, there is no *withdrawal* of treatment from him until a further acute change occurs in his condition. This change took place on the evening of day seven, when John suffers a reoccurrence of gastro-intestinal bleeding, and develops a serious cardiac arrhythmia. He suffers further bleeding across the course of day eight, and the accompanying atrial fibrillation becomes intractable. On the afternoon of day nine, after John's wife has been contacted and has arrived to be with him, the cardiac drugs he is receiving are switched off and his oxygen reduced. He dies shortly afterwards.

The trajectory of John's death is relatively slow. Negotiation takes place across the course of several days and there is a gradual movement from 'full' treatment, to withholding treatment, and then finally to 'withdrawal'. The latter only occurs when it becomes clear that death will occur *in spite of* any further treatment manoeuvres. In this way a causative link between non-treatment and death is avoided, and 'bodily' death is aligned to 'technical' death. So it is that 'natural' death is successfully constructed.

The next example demonstrates the problems of constructing 'natural death' in a situation where a much more rapid, acute bodily deterioration occurs. The data discussed here are drawn from the case of 'Richard', a young man who had been fatally injured in a road traffic accident and who died after seven days in intensive care.

Balancing medical action and non-action: Richard's case

In Richard's case, 'bodily' death threatens to *outpace* the evolving process of negotiation that is necessary to confirm 'technical' death and to allow treatment withdrawal to precede bodily death. In this situation, particular efforts are employed to ensure the 'balancing' of medical action and the distribution of responsibility between members of the medical team, and between them and Richard's body. It is noteworthy that this case involves a much younger man, who had previously been fully fit. His youth and 'fitness' appear to play a large part in the reluctance to stop medical treatment.

We join Richard's case on the morning of day seven, just over six hours before his death. The previous afternoon there had been a sudden and severe deterioration in his condition due to internal bleeding. I arrive in the unit at 08:45. The senior registrar and the registrar are in the staff room and I speak to them, asking how Richard is:

> *The senior registrar shakes his head: 'Dreadful, dreadful.'*

> *I go through to the unit and the senior registrar follows, speaking to me: 'Have you seen his face yet today?' The curtains are around the bed. I say that no, I haven't.*

> *Senior Registrar: 'Well, he looks dead, I mean he is dead to all intents and purposes – but I can't do anything yet – we've tried reducing the vasopressin to give him a bit more peripheral perfusion, but his colour is still just awful -- you press his skin, it blanches and then very, very sluggishly there is some colour, but it's a blue-yellow colour rather than red. I'm going to have to wait until Consultant C does his round, and then we've got to step back from this.'*
>
> (From the field notes, day 7)

Richard, in the ordinary 'bodily' sense, has died, but in this 'extraordinary' environment, it becomes the responsibility of the medical staff to 'allow' this to happen on the basis of a technical definition. The medical hierarchy that exists means that the senior registrar cannot act on what he sees and what he feels to be true; he must wait for the duty consultant to legitimate this.

Over the next few hours activity continues around Richard in much the same way as the other patients. However, the faces of the staff as they work are grim and they are almost silent.

Consultant C arrives at 12:15. He immediately telephones the surgical consultant to come and see Richard. The exchange that follows shows how the consultant surgeon and consultant anaesthetist communicate their definition of Richard's condition to each other through an exploration of the boundaries of their individual responsibilities, and the part that Richard himself has had to play in events. The exchange ends with a re-working of the situation, not as failure, but as the best that could have been achieved in the circumstances:

> *Consultant C (to the surgeon): 'Our major problem is that he has a severe metabolic acidosis with a ph of 6.9. and a base excess of –26, [showing cellular hypoxia] in spite of everything we are doing and in spite of a normal PO_2 [arterial pressure of oxygen].'*
> *Surgeon: 'Why do you think he has gone off then?'*
> *Consultant C: 'Well it's basically to do with shunting -- we can deliver the oxygen to him but he is not able to use it and so the body organs gradually die off.'*
> *Surgeon: 'If there was a surgical cause -- if by decompressing his abdomen that would make a difference, then I would be prepared to intervene, but from what you are saying it will not do so?'*

Consultant C: 'Well, no, his abdomen is more distended, but he will die if we take him and he will die if we leave him like this anyway for a day or so. I will of course look at everything this afternoon, X-rays, blood results, etc, but I really think we have to accept that he is not going to survive and make a decision to take his drive [cardiac drugs] off. The relatives are not here at the moment, so we will have to wait.'

Surgeon: 'Well, it's just a tragic case. All you can do with such a young man is everything you can think of. You've done well to keep him alive for a week -- not that it is of any comfort I don't suppose.'

(From the field notes, day 7)

The consultant presents the 'problem' as belonging to the intensive care medical staff describing it in complex physiological terms. In asking for clarification: ('why has he gone off then?') the surgeon relocates the 'problem' as belonging to Richard. The consultant responds by drawing the boundary around the expectations that can be held of his treatment: 'We can deliver the oxygen to him, but he is not able to use it.' Having checked that surgical intervention will not improve the situation, the surgeon acquiesces to the proposal to withdraw Richard's cardiac drugs and then quickly offers a definition of the situation that supports the actions taken over the last week as '*all*' that could have been done: 'You've done well to keep him alive for a week'. With his family sitting beside him, Richard's drugs are switched off. He dies five minutes later, seven days after his accident.

Discussion

In this chapter the various elements involved in the definition and management of 'dying' during the accomplishment of medical work in intensive care have been delineated. It has been suggested that clinicians negotiate 'natural' death in intensive care by means of complex interactional strategies in which the timing of treatment withdrawal is carefully planned, and is accompanied by expressions of belief about the causation of death and the distribution of responsibility for decision making between clinicians, patients, nurses and family members. The existence has been highlighted of two potentially divergent dying trajectories, 'technical' and 'bodily' dying, which must be aligned in order for death to occur at the 'right' time. Containing and preventing divergence between bodily and technical dying are represented as the basis of 'nature taking its course' and 'natural death' in intensive care.

Intensive care reflects the modern preoccupation with the mastery of disease and the eradication of 'untimely death'. It is the place to which clinicians may refer a patient when that individual stands at the brink of death and is beyond the reach of conventional therapies. Unravelling the nature of complex disease and predicting its outcome is complicated by a lack of previous familiarity between healthcare staff and the patient, by the unconscious state of the ill person (Muller and Koenig 1988), and by the advanced technical abilities of modern medicine to blur the boundaries between living and dying. Further, it is acknowledged that in spite of efforts to diminish any distinction between withholding and withdrawing treatments (BMA 1999), the process of withdrawing treatments once instituted is emotionally fraught and subject to many difficulties. At the centre of this are debates about the proper role of medicine and medical practitioners at the end of life, and a current climate in which most doctors are keen to distance themselves from any actions that might be interpreted as active euthanasia (Johnston and Pfeifer 1998). At the same time, an argument has been developed (Hopkins 1997), which suggests that withdrawing treatments, in order that a recognized process of dying may replace any artificial prolongation of life, is morally no different to active euthanasia:[2]

> In looking at actions which count as 'passive' and which actually count as 'active' it is clear that the practice of euthanasia consistently revolves around notions of a 'natural' death, the 'natural' course of disease, and the contextual permissibility of 'unplugging machines' and 'withdrawing treatments'. Subtly but crucially evident in these concerns is a conceptual reliance on a form of the nature/culture distinction – the distinction between the 'natural' and the 'artificial' – and on particular assumptions about the definition and moral relevance of technology.
>
> (Hopkins 1997: 29)

The answer to the question of why individual patients frequently receive protracted and costly multiple organ system support in the hours and days immediately before death (Faber-Langendoen and Bartels 1992; Singer 1994; Principal Investigators for the SUPPORT Project 1995; Bion and Strunin 1996; Faber-Langendoen 1996), even when death is recognized as certain, lies it would seem, within this paradox of what constitutes 'natural' and 'artificial' in a highly technologized society at the start of its third millennium. It is recognized increasingly that most deaths are managed in some way (Ashby 1998); what we lack is knowledge about the process of that management with which to inform and improve care at the end of life.

Focusing on the intricacies of social interaction in the specialized environment of intensive care helps to shed light on the way in which the paradox of 'natural' and 'artificial' is dealt with at the bedside and how the disparate understandings of medical science and clinical wisdom are reconciled. Further, an analytical framework has been presented, which may be of value in elucidating the complex processes that underpin the deferral of death and dying in high technology areas of health care. The difficulties that clinicians face during the course of their everyday work with critically ill and dying people must be allowed to further inform our thinking about the 'modern myth' of natural death (Hopkins 1997) if 'death with dignity' is to become a reality in our healthcare systems. As Ashby notes, until better understanding is reached and greater debate encouraged about the management of end-of-life care, it will remain the case that clinical behaviour will range from: 'abrupt cessation of treatment, minimalist palliative care and treatment directed at bringing about a rapid dying process, to excessive caution about being seen to be instrumental in causing the death' (1998: 74).

Notes

1 This emphasis on problems of definition between treatment withdrawal, euthanasia and 'natural death' may give the impression that medical action was *always* conscious, purposive and explicit in its approach to overcoming these distinctions. I do not think this was always the case: such problems of definition were habitually dealt with, and only became problematic in certain situations.
2 This philosophical argument hinges on a particular conception of causation. Hopkins argues that the withdrawal of artificial treatments (as opposed to the underlying disease process) *causes* death, and therefore there is no difference between withdrawal of such treatments and the administration of an artificial treatment (such as a drug) designed to achieve euthanasia. For a detailed discussion of causality and its role in end-of-life decision making see Ashby (1998).

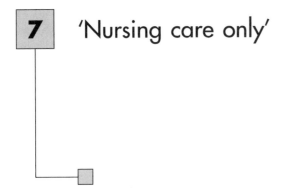

7 'Nursing care only'

This chapter examines the problematic constitution of 'nursing care only' within intensive care and expands on the description of nursing work presented in Chapter 4. There the discussion focused on the identification of the contingent and contradictory aspects of nursing in intensive care, with a suggestion that nurses' actions are determined primarily by the medically framed aspects of their role. This chapter examines the tensions that further attend nursing as medical treatment is withdrawn and patients enter a phase known as 'nursing care only'.[1] The alignment of 'body work' (Lawler 1991) with 'emotional work' (Hochschild 1983; James 1989, 1992; Smith 1992) is posited in this chapter as a central element of nursing work with dying people in the medically framed, 'decontextualised and technologised' (Kastenbaum and Aisenberg 1972: 207) area of intensive care. Such 'work' means that it becomes possible to reproduce subjectivity within the apparently lifeless form of each individual and to relocate death and dying from the biomedical sphere to the arena of emotion and familial intimacy. In this way, nurses fashion their work with dying people in intensive care, investing meaning and purpose into a potentially contradictory aspect of their role.

'Knowing the patient': a background

Tanner *et al.* (1993), writing about nursing knowledge in intensive care, trace a development that takes place during the acquisition of nursing expertise. This results in the discourse of 'knowing the patient' and is defined as:

> a reference to how they [nurses] understood the patient, grasped the meaning of the situation for the patient, or recognized the need for a

particular action. In expert nursing practice this kind of knowing is very different from the formalized, explicit, decontextualized data-based knowledge that constitutes formal assessments, yet it is central to skilled nursing judgement.

(Tanner *et al.* 1993: 73)

While the trend in medicine is to subsume 'knowing the patient' to the formal rationality of science, the discourse of the 'informal' has become incorporated into the very essence of the ideology of caring and compassion within nursing. One aspect of this has been identified by post-structuralist authors such as Armstrong (1983b) and May (1992a,b). They examine the concept of 'knowing the patient' in their analyses of the incorporation of 'the social' into nursing work in non-intensive care areas. For such authors, 'knowing the patient' depends on the *conversational* practices with conscious, interacting patients. Through these practices the clinical 'gaze', which investigates and invigilates the body (Foucault 1976), is extended to a 'subjective' or 'therapeutic' gaze (Bloor and McIntosh 1990) in which 'the patient' is constituted as a 'whole' psycho-social being. May, in his analysis of the process of nursing terminally ill patients, has suggested that the incorporation of the 'subjective' into nursing has had the effect of creating a social expectation of 'unproblematic dying' in which individuals: 'die without pain, and are able to convey their feelings to near relatives and friends; (but) also having resolved private fears and anxieties' (May 1992a: 595).

Here, May suggests, nurses' attention shifts from the 'concrete condition of the body' (1992a: 591) towards the patient's subjective sphere. In making this distinction between 'body work' and 'subjective work', May draws on research which shows that in practice, while nurses are aware of patients' psychosocial needs, they seem to concentrate frequently on the tasks associated with physical care-giving (Peterson 1988). May concludes from this that, while it is the case that nursing *discourse* is increasingly oriented around individuals, nursing *action* is constrained by a range of structural and organizational constraints, which make the aspirations encapsulated in such discourse difficult to attain (see, for example, Field 1989; James and Field 1996). Moreover, as May argues, drawing on his own research (1991) and that of Lawler (1991) and Handy (1991), the ability of nurses to 'assemble and recognise patients as subjects' (May 1992a: 595) is set on shaky foundations. It may be challenged at any moment by patients' exercise of the option to 'remain silent' (Bloor and McIntosh 1990).

Clearly, 'conversational' practices leading to apprehension of subjectivity are not available for nurses working with dying people within intensive care because of the lack of opportunities to have verbal interaction with patients. At first sight, then, this presents a significant difficulty for nurses in their attempts to enact the 'new holism' of nursing (Lupton 1995).

However, as we saw in Chapter 4, caring for the 'whole person' remains central to the way in which nurses perceive, and account for, their work in intensive care.

The intensive care literature sheds some light on this paradox, suggesting that nurses develop 'knowing in action' (Schön 1983) or 'embodied knowledge' (Benner and Wrubel 1989) in which physical care-giving and the delivery of emotional and psychosocial care are intertwined. Benner and Wrubel argue that this means that experienced intensive care nurses are able to respond in an intuitively expert way to the subjective needs of their patients *even* when that individual is unable to communicate verbally. They argue that in this way nurses develop intimate relationships with their patients and are able to respond to them in an almost familial way. Developing this argument, Benner and colleagues (Benner *et al.* 1996) suggest that emotional involvement is a key aspect of 'understanding', and of responding appropriately to, the patient and the patient's family. Writing about a particular clinical anecdote they say this:

> [the nurse] understood the past for this patient, had an immediate clinical grasp of the present crisis, and could project to the future. Because of this understanding, the nurse could help the family anticipate what lay ahead . . . for this nurse, the patient is no longer a medical case, but a person with a life full of meaning. She is engaged emotionally with his life world . . . this emotional involvement makes it possible for her to respond to the family in a sensitive and meaningful way.
>
> (Benner *et al.* 1996: 7–8)

Some commentators suggest that the exhortation to introduce an overtly emotional component into nursing work in intensive care has led to a situation of 'moral distress' (Rodney 1988; Corley 1995) in which the primary experiences are of powerlessness *vis à vis* medicine, and a sense of anger, sadness and frustration during the care of dying patients (Yarling and McElmurry 1986; Erlan and Frost 1991). Degner and Beaton's four-year study of life and death decisions in acute care settings in Canada (1987) suggests that nurses' conceptualization of their work leads frequently to disagreements with medical staff over the continuation of treatment for patients:

> Nurses are . . . upset by treatment decisions with which they do not agree, particularly when the nurses are the ones who have to implement the decision. Aggressive treatment that nurses think is unwarranted provokes the most intense resentment . . . although not totally powerless in such situations, nurses do find themselves carrying out orders with which they disagree and over which they have little control.
>
> (Degner and Beaton 1987: 22)

As we have seen, however, nurses do not always express such disagreements openly. Rather they subvert and cloak their feelings in order that the medical work of assembling a case to justify 'technical dying' is not disrupted. Shedding light on this observation, James (1989, 1992) describes eloquently how the expression of emotion associated with nursing work is attended frequently by contradiction since, when unregulated and expressed freely, it does not fit in with expectations of what should occur at work nor with standard ideas of work skills. Developing the work of Hochschild (1983) James employs the term 'emotional labour' to account for the manner in which nurses manage emotions in such a way as to avoid disruption to the normal work routines of their particular working environment. Emotional labour, suggests James, acts as a form of regulation of emotional expression yet also, paradoxically, facilitates the emotional expression that is so necessary for the accomplishment of 'good' nursing. Giving insight into the 'emotional labour' undertaken by nurses in intensive care, Simpson (1997) describes how nurses use emotional expression as a means of overcoming 'the dehumanizing aspects of dying in a technological environment' (1997: 189), and to allow the 'reconnection' of patients with their families. Simpson argues that this process of reconnection, in which emotional expression and investment by nurses plays such an important role, underpins the breakdown of barriers between the dying person and his or her companions, *and* plays a central role in the development of trust between companions and clinical staff. Simpson implies that bodily care, which she calls 'basic care', is an integral aspect of 'reconnection' by means of which nurses are able to prepare families for the death of the patient: 'Basic care was continued to ensure that the patient was well cared for, again as much for the benefit of the family as the patient. The nurses attempted to provide privacy for the family, to answer their questions and to 'be there' for the family' (1997: 195).

We turn now to see how nurses in this study managed the twin demands of reproducing subjectivity and managing emotions during their care of dying patients in intensive care. The discussion begins by showing how 'bodily work' is an integral part of emotional expression within the intensive care environment, and how nurses engender subjectivity within the bodies of dying patients during, and perhaps as a result of, the fastidious and compassionate bodily care they deliver. Alongside this primary focus, nursing work is shown to be directed also towards the creation of an atmosphere of intimacy and familial warmth during the process of death. Here, very significant efforts are expended in encouraging family members to be with the dying person. Attention then turns to how nurses manage 'nursing care only' against the backdrop of the potentially divergent trajectories of bodily and technical dying highlighted in the last chapter. The problems of reproducing subjectivity and managing technology during delayed bodily dying are particularly highlighted.

Aligning bodily and emotional work during dying

For some critically ill individuals in this study, medical treatment was finally withdrawn moments before their death. As described in Chapter 6, in such cases bodily death had usually begun to occur before an agreement had been reached concerning the removal of medical treatment and the definition of technical death. In other cases, the trajectory of bodily death lagged behind the removal of medical treatment and definition of technical death. Death took longer to occur and the care of the dying person was openly acknowledged to be the province of the nursing staff. In spite of these differences, a common feature of all cases was the subtle change in emphasis towards those individuals 'known' to be dying in a 'technical' sense, and those 'seen' to be dying in a 'bodily' sense.

A repeated feature of the observational data in this research was the pre-eminence of painstaking physical care on the part of the nursing staff. Some general observations will be made here concerning this. During the case of 'Mr Hart', who had suffered a severe head injury, and was recognized as dying at an early stage in his treatment, very considerable efforts were made by the nursing staff to ensure that he looked clean and comfortable. His wife later remembered:

> them really caring for him as though he was going to be alright, you know what I mean, they didn't treat him just like someone who wasn't going to make it and they weren't going to bother; they really cared for him and washed him and turned him . . . they treated him like he was a patient who was going to be alright.
>
> (From follow-up interview)

This treatment of the dying Mr Hart seems to comfort his wife because, for her, it represents an acknowledgement of his social significance. Similarly the careful attention to Mr Hart's bodily needs and appearance is construed by his son, Michael, as an act of respect normally preserved for those people who are 'expected to live':

> everyone treated him with the respect that you would with someone who'd just gone under a normal operation and who was going to wake up sooner or later
>
> (From follow-up interview)

This preservation, or reproduction of social presence, was further encouraged by the nursing staff through the development of an intimate relationship with Mrs Hart and with Michael. Thus I observed how they encouraged Mrs Hart to reinforce her husband's social presence by reminiscing aloud and by showing photographs of him. They also encouraged Michael and Mrs Hart to sit beside him and to refer repeatedly to what *he* would have wished had he been able to make his wishes known. These practices imbued

Mr Hart's death with a sense of familial intimacy and emotional warmth. In my interpretation, what was occurring here was an alignment of 'body work' with 'emotional work' such that the 'whole person' of Mr Hart could be reproduced.

In this example such alignment was apparently successful. In other cases, the alignment was very much more difficult to sustain. For instance, in the case of Richard Morgan, the young man discussed in Chapter 6, medical treatment is not withdrawn until after profound changes in bodily appearance, indicative of imminent death, take place. This poses a problem for the nurse who is looking after him on that day. She described later how:

> we had to continue making up all his drips, washing him and cleaning, just doing the usual care that you give to other patients but I knew by looking at him, . . . it was like 'Why am I doing this?' I knew I was doing it because they hadn't decided to withdraw but I just wanted to get someone in to look at him and say to them: 'How would you like your relative to look like this?' and: 'You're doing all this treatment but you're not doing anything'.
>
> (From follow-up interview)

In Richard's case, the dissonance between the requirement to care for his 'already dead' body and ideology of 'whole person' seems to be solved by an attribution to Richard of particular personal qualities. Thus it becomes possible for the nurse to describe him as 'fighting', as 'still living' and later:

> he was strong and trying to say: 'I'm not giving up' although his body was saying: 'You can't survive with this,' I felt his heart and his brain was fighting everything
>
> (From follow-up interview)

In her attribution to Richard of agency and intentionality, this nurse makes an almost Cartesian distinction between the appearance of his obviously dying body and her sense of his 'person' as something that exists *outside* of the disintegrating, unresponsive body for which she was having to care. In so doing, she apprehends his personhood successfully and achieves a sense of meaning in her work, albeit at considerable personal cost. She recalled how his image remained in her mind long after his death:

> JS: Does that memory stick out more in your mind than say, some other patients that you've looked after in the previous 2 years 9 months? [length of time she had worked in intensive care].
> *Nurse*: Yes, Richard, really, I was -- erm -- I couldn't stop thinking about him. I can still see him.
>
> (From follow-up interview)

Another aspect of her care was an attempt to pre-warn and 'prepare' his family for his imminent death. This, however, was fraught with difficulty because, for them, the apparent continuation of 'full medical treatment', conjoined with his long period of unconsciousness, obscures the material fact of death. In her follow-up interview the nurse remembers them as being 'devastated' by the eventual formal news given to them by the Consultant. She believes that they misconstrued the activities around Richard as a sign of continuing hope of recovery.

In other cases, nurses resolved the dissonance described above by a determined relocation of emotional work to the ill person's companions. In such situations the physical care of the ill person was no less fastidious, but the attribution of personal qualities and characteristics was absent. Instead, what seemed to occur was an attempt to engender the subjectivity of the ill person through the production of an appropriate emotional response within their companions. The cases described in Chapter 5 concerning Mr Smith, and Mr Oldham capture this. There we saw the attempts to bring Mary, Mr Smith's wife, to 'open awareness' of his impending death, and the problems perceived by the nurses when Mrs Oldham feels unable to sit beside her husband.

We now turn to the enactment of 'nursing care only' both in those situations where there was open acknowledgement of 'technical' death, and in those where the definition of 'technical' death was delayed. Material from three case examples will be used to delineate the range of problematic issues involved. The first concerns the struggle of one nurse to 'manage' the dying and death of a man whose imminent 'technical death' had been confirmed the day before she arrives to take over his care for the 'early shift'. The focus in this example is the attempt of the nurse to reproduce the subjectivity of the dying man during the protracted process of his bodily dying and her interpretation of the meaning of her involvement with him and his wife. The second examines a contrasting situation in which a definition of 'technical death' was delayed. As in the first, the focus here is on the manoeuvres of one particular nurse as she attempts to engage in a range of 'caring' activities around the 'bodily' dying woman concerned. The third example focuses more closely on the potential conflicts between nurses as they manage the residual technology surrounding a dying woman from whom active medical treatment had been withdrawn. This example shows the uncertainties and risks that emerge as nursing moves into the 'semantic space' (May 1992b) vacated by medicine.

Reproducing subjectivity and meaning in nursing work

Mr Albert Randall had been admitted to the intensive care unit at Western Hospital following surgery for a perforated duodenal ulcer. Mr Randall's case was introduced in Chapter 3. Here we rejoin the situation the day after it had been decided by medical staff that 'active treatment' would no longer be given. It is the general shift handover from the night staff to the 'early' staff. The charge-nurse, Z, who has been caring for Mr Randall overnight, is speaking:

> Z: 'We've turned him about three times, his feed is still going and he's on ten breaths [of the ventilator]. I didn't adjust the ventilator down any more, because I think he would go quickly, and I didn't think it was fair to 'phone his wife at 3 or 4 o'clock in the morning.'

At the bedside Z hands over in more detail to Nurse A and they talk about how best to manage his death:

> A: 'What do you think I should do Z? Should I, am I allowed to take his et. [endo-tracheal] tube out?'
> Z: 'No you can't, but boy, did I want to. I think it looks gross ... I really wish we could get it out and make him look really nice for his wife. We can't take it out without the doctors' say so though.'
> A: 'What about 'phoning his wife, when should I do that?'
> Z: 'Well, if I were you, I'd wait until about 09:00 and then put him on a "t" piece, turn off the pressure support [accepted techniques of reducing respiratory support in what is known as a "terminal wean" situation], and then call his wife – it won't be long then.'

(From the field notes)

Nurse A is left at this point to try to carry through these plans. The following section examines the way in which she attempted to do this, while simultaneously being required to carry out the more medically led plans for Mr Randall, focusing particularly on the account she gave of the events in her follow-up interview.

After the charge-nurse Z leaves, Nurse A is left alone to look after Mr Randall. She speaks to another nurse and to myself (I have been listening to the bedside handover) about her plans: she says that she has decided to wait until Mrs Randall phones the unit, rather than telephoning Mrs Randall herself. She voices the hope that he will stay 'stable' in the meantime, and says that she will not put him on a 't' piece until she hears that Mrs Randall is on her way to the hospital. She makes ready to wash Mr Randall, drawing the curtains around the bed:

> A: 'I'm going to make a start and get him washed and looking good, so that when she does ring, we're all ready.'

(From the field notes, day 10)

Having drawn these plans, events do not unfold in the way that A expects, and she becomes increasingly anxious. Mrs Randall does not telephone the unit as A hopes. Then she is asked by the medical staff to remove the ventilator from Mr Randall. A attempts to contact Mrs Randall before she takes the ventilator away, and gets no reply to her call. She eventually takes Mr Randall off the ventilator at 11:30, without his wife being present. She carefully ensures that he is breathing comfortably without the ventilator, adjusting the tubing attached to his endo-tracheal tube to ensure that there is no obstruction to the flow of air. I realize that she is upset and decide to leave in order to avoid adding to her stress:

When the ventilator has been removed, A carefully checks Mr Randall to make sure he is comfortable. He flickers his eyes and moves slightly and she talks reassuringly to him. She starts to write her report, head bent and avoiding eye contact with anyone. Other nurses keep coming and asking her to keep an 'eye' on their patients (who are deemed more in need of attention because they are more 'sick'?) while they get drugs or have a break. I go over to tell her that I will leave after the pm handover and wait while she finishes writing. I start to speak and then realize that she is very, very distressed. I ask her if she is OK and she starts to cry – I put my arm around her, and she tells me that she is feeling very unhappy:

'I can't get hold of his wife and I really think that he might die without her being here. I think she ought to have the opportunity to come in. Now I've been told to take him off of the vent, and I really feel like I am killing him -- I think it's partly because I looked after him the other day and I felt he was responding a bit to me, and even now, he's flinching at times --' She cries more.

I try to reassure her, that she has tried her best to contact Mrs Randall and how comfortable he looks. I apologize that I cannot do anything to help her sort the situation out but advise her that she needs to talk to the nurse in charge. She is reluctant to do this, but allows me to speak to the 'f' grade staff nurse. I do this as tactfully as I can, and then return with some tissues for her. She is calmer now, and I get my bag ready to leave.

As I am leaving. I see the 'f' grade taking A into the 'quiet' room, she nods at me. A is crying again.

(From the field notes, day 10)

One month after these events I am able to interview A about her recollections. She gives an account of why the situation was so difficult for her, explaining it in terms of her intimate 'knowledge' about Mr Randall 'himself', her desire to achieve the 'right' kind of death for him, and her lack of understanding about, and control of, the process of decision making surrounding his death. She starts her account by explaining how 'depressed' she was that Mr Randall had been transferred eventually to a ward (rather than dying on intensive care):

A: the thing that really got me lately was Mr Randall; you know about him anyway. The thing that really got me there was at the end of the shift they transferred him to the ward and -- I don't know, -- that was the hardest thing I've had to deal with on here because it was depressing. I didn't feel like I was getting anywhere, it was just depressing.

JS: Can you tell me what it was like for you when you were involved in his care?

A: Well, I'd actually looked after him the previous week on nights and came back onto days and looked after him again. That was my choice. I wanted to do it because I felt like he knew me; because now and again he would open his eyes, and I just wanted to be there for him. I wanted him to know that I was there. I think also, that dying patients, some nurses don't let them know that they are there, just by, you know, touch, holding his hand, stuff like this, and I wanted to do that, just so as he knew that he wasn't on his own. His wife didn't want to be there -- although I didn't know that until the day I thought he was actually going to die. So I don't know, I felt like the pressure was on me. His wife didn't want to be there, I'd tried to contact her, I'd said to her the previous night: 'If you go out tomorrow, leave me a number' and she didn't. So it was obvious that she didn't want to come in. I just felt like I was -- I don't know -- the only person he'd got. Do you know what I mean? To sort of see him out . . . and he reminded me of my granddad (slight embarrassed laugh) as well. And the fact he was an alcoholic. When I'd looked after him on nights, someone said, 'Oh, yeah, he's an alcoholic, and he's needed heminevrin down on the ward', and that sort of blackens your view; and yet, when it came to it and I'd spoken to his wife, it turns out that he wasn't like that at all; he might have been like it in hospital when he was ill, but at home he used to go down and help these homeless people who were alcoholic as well. You know, he did a lot of good work. I thought, bloody hell, I've thought badly of you, and I shouldn't have done at all . . . I just felt so sorry for him, he looked so childish lying there and he had his eyes open now and again, and I thought, 'Christ, I ought to be telling him he's dying, does he know?' In case there was anything he wanted to say – he probably couldn't speak, but maybe mouth something . . . they'd already withdrawn when I came on duty that day, but what got me was that he was a bit more with it and I just thought, are they doing the right thing?

(From follow-up interview)

A's ideal of death is revealed here – physical contact with a close, 'known' individual, facilitation of communication, knowledge of imminent dying. She interprets Mrs Randall's absence in a particular way, feeling that the burden to achieve this sort of death then falls on her shoulders alone. Her memory of her grandfather further forges a sense of connection with Mr Randall and imbues her relationship with him with a sense of intimacy, so much so that she requests to be allowed to care for him. This ideal death, for her, must also be intelligible according to, as she sees it, her 'basic' understanding of medicine, and yet this is not so: she remembers not understanding why the withdrawal of treatment is being carried out, and not being provided with the explanations that she needs to make sense of events:

> Er, the thing is, because you think, feel, that the doctors know every-thing, I'd said to them, look, well, he's more, well, he seemed more with it neurologically, and even one of the doctors thought that as well. I think he had second thoughts about withdrawing, and you think Christ, if he [the doctor] is, why don't they try and start to treat him again . . . if a doctor thinks that he might make it, then, you know. But they still didn't . . . maybe they could have explained things a bit better to people like me, I mean I've got a basic understanding, so if they'd explained it better then maybe I could've coped with it better myself, you know.
>
> (From follow-up interview)

Thus for A, her work with Mr Randall becomes a source of stressful contradiction: her ideal of what constitutes nursing care for a dying person means that she sets the task for herself of 'being there for him' as he dies. She indeed achieves a particular sense of closeness to him, imagining that he is a 'known' person, much like her own, loved grandfather. She takes on the burden of trying to engender a situation where his wife is 'with him' and close to him, and finds it incomprehensible when Mrs Randall does not respond in the way she expects. When she has to carry out what to her is the final, illogical withdrawal of technological support; all of the intimacy that she has crafted so carefully is compromised. She recalls that: '*I suppose I felt like I was killing him*', and, with his transfer out of intensive care to be nursed by strangers, the connection is finally broken between herself and Mr Randall.

This situation involved the struggles of a relatively inexperienced nurse who was attempting to deliver 'nursing' to a man from whom medical attention had been withdrawn formally. The next example looks at the way in which a very much more experienced nurse negotiated the delivery of 'nursing' to a dying woman who had not yet been designated formally as 'for nursing care only'. Here behind the scenes negotiations were still in progress about the formal acknowledgement of dying. These exchanges were between the intensive care medical staff and the surgical staff who had admitted the woman to hospital. We have here a clear example of 'seen bodily death' outpacing 'known technical death'.

Negotiating 'nursing' in a situation of delayed 'technical' death

We rejoin Mrs Hall's case the day after an interview between her family and the senior registrar in which they are warned about a possible withdrawal of treatment. The events leading up to this situation were described in Chapter 4.

The morning after the interview considerable concern is expressed by the nursing staff about what the response of the family was when they were interviewed. The nurses G and Y read the information sheet closely, trying to assess what the likely effect would have been. G is Mrs Hall's named nurse but has not looked after her for two days. There is no one on duty who was present during the interview. The senior registrar and the consultant who were on duty yesterday are not available this morning; another consultant will be in charge of the unit for the morning. The night staff nurse, who is handing over the care of Mrs Hall to G and Y, says she has had a 'phone-call from one of Mrs Hall's sons. She reports that he has asked: 'how long have I got before she dies?' and: 'should I go to work or not?' The night staff nurse has had to evade giving a direct answer, because she is aware that until the cardiovascular drugs are turned off Mrs Hall could survive for days. She has advised him to come in during the course of the morning, however. G is particularly concerned that no analgesia or sedation other than intra-muscular haloperidol has been given to Mrs Hall. The field notes record my impressions at this time:

> *Little Mrs Hall – she is a tiny frail lady – lies quivering slightly – eyes tightly shut. Difficult to tell if she is aware or not. Her left foot moves up and down on the pillow it is resting on.*
>
> *G and Y are busy taking blood, labelling and bagging it. Doing observations and measuring urine. G goes to get all the 9 am drugs and as she returns the duty reg. from last night is handing over to the new duty reg. Last night's reg. looks desperately tired and obviously has to concentrate hard to give a reasonable account of Mrs Hall.*
>
> *One registrar says to the other: 'This is a bit of a half way house isn't it? Either we dialyze her or we stop – that's the way I see it anyway.' G looks up from beside Mrs Hall and says wryly: 'You're not the only one!'*
>
> (From the field notes)

Thus we have a picture of a desperately sick, dying person surrounded by staff who know she is going to die but are carrying out the various procedures and tasks usually involved in caring for those people who are not expected to die. The shared discomfort of the nurses and the registrars is apparent, as they wait for the duty consultant to do his ward round. What happens next is a stark example, I would suggest, of a particular pattern of dissent and conflict surrounding the delivery of nursing care and medical treatment to Mrs Hall. Until now, that conflict has been successfully 'cloaked' but now becomes more openly expressed.

The duty consultant arrives as the registrars finish their exchange next to Mrs Hall's bed. He looks at Mrs Hall and says to the assembled staff: '*This is the lady from last week isn't it?*' (It is a Monday morning and this consultant has not been on the unit since Friday morning.) Nurse G is rather scathing in her reply: '*Wow! You're on the ball today!*' She tells me later that this is her way of 'telling off' doctors who are 'too lazy to remember people'. The consultant seems to take this as a purely humorous remark and, after reading the brief entries written in the notes by the senior registrar and Consultant 1 from yesterday, asks G to tell him what has been happening since Friday. He directs his request to G rather than to the registrars who are standing next to him, almost as if G will be able to give him a more reliable overall account. G however rejects this request:

> Nurse G: '*It's all written down Doc.*'
> Consultant: '*Can't you just give me a summary?*'
> Nurse G: (*nodding very meaningfully towards Mrs Hall, i.e. she can probably hear.*) '*No.*'
> The consultant realizes what Nurse G is trying to tell him and goes back to reading the notes. He flicks to the relatives' information sheet and reads. After a while he looks up and says: '*OK, that's very clear. Have the physicians been involved over the weekend?*'
> (From the field notes)

The physicians referred to here are the team under which Mrs Hall was admitted the week before. The registrar tells Consultant 2 that there has been no involvement with them over the last few days. Nonetheless Consultant 2 decides that the consultant physician, Doctor W, must be contacted:

> '*Well, what I shall do is 'phone Dr W and discuss with him what it is best to do. I think we all know what we think is best, but this has to be a joint decision between us, the physician and the family. So I will liaise with you, G, . . . when I've spoken to him and then we sort out what to stop and about sedation and everything.*'
> (From the field notes)

Nurse G asks him what she should do about the antibiotics that Mrs Hall is receiving. He asks her to carry on giving them:

> '*Until I've spoken to Dr W we've got to press on.*'
> (From the field notes)

The impression gained from observing this piece of interaction was that the consultant could very much decide on the course of action to be taken with little reference to the other staff. He had appealed to nurse G to provide him with information, but she had not been willing to do this, implying that Mrs Hall would be able to hear what was said. There also seemed to be an element of resignation: 'It's all written down Doc', as if the entries in the medical notes were the information he was likely to take as most reliable. G does not leave her position beside Mrs Hall to engage in a more formal conversation with the consultant, and the exchange seems almost casual, with G periodically making remarks to Y, her nursing colleague, and busying herself attending to the multitude of observations, and drug infusions that Mrs Hall is still receiving. Likewise, the registrar proffers information only in response to a direct question. She does not voice her earlier misgivings: 'This is a bit of a half-way house, isn't it', to the consultant.

Nurse G becomes increasingly impatient and anxious during the course of the morning. Consultant 2 moves away to attend to another patient and then a new admission arrives, which absorbs his time over the next few hours. At one point G comes across to me (I am standing by the nurses' station), and I ask her what is happening:

> *She tells me that she is still waiting. She is angry and upset, although resigned: 'He (Cons 2) hasn't got hold of Dr W yet. He says that it's because Dr W is in clinic. Now if I were them I would have 'phoned him anyway and said: 'Look – this is the situation, are you in agreement with our plans?' It's not as if Dr W doesn't know Mrs Hall. Meanwhile I'm left feeling really bad having to put up more antibiotics and stuff that I don't think I should be giving any more. Now usually I tell the patient and their family exactly what I'm doing, but because I feel so stupid, I didn't say anything at 12:00. Of course they (the family) looked at me as much as to say, G, what are you doing, she's dying isn't she?'*

> *I ask her why she does not feel able to tell them.*

> G: *'I suppose I'm embarrassed – I mean they were more or less told yesterday at four o'clock that a final decision would be taken this morning, but that basically she wasn't going to make it, and now its 1 pm and they've been here since 10:30 and nothing has happened.'*
>
> (From the field notes)

Shortly after this conversation Consultant 1 (who had been on call over the weekend) arrives. G says to me: '*Good, he'll probably get the diamorphine going.*' The reference to diamorphine is significant because the drug is almost always used to ensure analgesia and sedation for those people who are 'formally' recognized as 'dying'. G sits down beside Consultant 1 at the nurses' station and starts to remonstrate with him. I cannot hear what is being said clearly, but pick up the general drift:

> *'What am I to say to her family? . . . I feel so awful putting up antibiotics . . . they've been here nearly four hours now waiting.'*

Consultant 1 looks harassed, and he is holding a phone up: 'Well, I've been trying to get hold of Dr W, but he wasn't to be disturbed this morning unless it was a matter of life or death . . .' G interrupts him: 'It is, someone is dying here!'

*Consultant 1: 'I **know**, but it's not an arrest or anything is it?'*

(From the field notes)

The exchange continues in slightly strained, although not unamicable tones. Eventually Consultant 1 gets heavily to his feet and agrees to go and have a look at Mrs Hall. Staff Nurse G reports to me (in her later interview) that no action was taken to reduce her treatment until several hours later:

Eventually Dr W was contacted and he agreed that we should let her die . . . but it was hours later.

JS: How did you feel when she did eventually die.

G: (small laugh) Relieved, if anything. I wasn't actually there when she did die, she died on the night shift and I was on the previous early, but relief for her and relief for the relatives I think. They probably didn't see it as this, but I knew, being a nurse and being on the inside if you like, I knew, that death could've been earlier. And hours earlier, I don't just mean a couple of hours, I mean quite a lot . . . even the night before, 12–24 hours earlier.

Long pause

JS: Did you feel that decision was taken at the wrong time?

G: Um . . . I think maybe the decision wasn't taken at the wrong time, I think it was a case of that before they made the decision or even before they spoke to the relatives they should have spoken to Dr W and said: 'Look, this is the situation', which is what normally happens, as far as I'm aware, so why it didn't happen in this case I don't know. There was something about Dr W being in clinic and there's no point interrupting his clinic unless it's a matter of life or death, and I took that literally, (slight laugh) and I said to the consultant: 'Well, actually, it's the latter isn't it?' and he just looked at me and smiled and said: 'Oh, yes, G the jolly one.' And I said: 'I'm being serious here! You're not taking me seriously.' And he said: 'Oh, well we'll just have to leave it here.'

(From follow-up interview)

Staff Nurse G thus clearly recollects her feelings at the time even though 10 weeks had passed. She reports her frustration at not 'being taken seriously,' and her difference of opinion with the consultant over what constituted an urgent 'life or death' situation. She goes on to tell me how these feelings of frustration affected her ability to support Mrs Hall's family who had gathered around their mother's bed. I too had observed how Mrs Hall's children and grandchildren had seemed puzzled by the continuing activities around her:

> Briefly there are six people around the bed. All the family bends close to Mrs Hall and kiss her. Then they sit quietly and anxiously, looking at the monitor, to the nurses and then back to Mrs Hall. G and Y are at the end of the bed and both look ill at ease and avoid eye contact with the family.

(From the field notes)

Staff Nurse G describes the situation of 'mutual pretense' that was perpetuated by the long delay in the process of withdrawing treatment from Mrs Hall and how this interfered with her stated wish to 'be there' for the family, with all the supportive intimacy this phrase implies:

> G: I found it very difficult to treat someone who was dying and we were still carrying on. They were looking at me, the relatives, while I was doing all these things as if to say: 'what are you doing?' But they never asked and I never said anything.
>
> JS: What do you think the impact on them was?'
>
> G: Well, I think -- um -- They knew what I was doing -- they didn't say anything, but you know the look that you can see as if to say, what are you doing? -- and (sighing) that was very difficult because I knew that they knew that I was still carrying on treating her.

(From follow-up interview)

The last case extract focuses on another complex problem involved in the enactment of 'nursing care only'. This concerns, first, the manipulation of the technological equipment that remains a feature of the management of dying in intensive care even when 'active' medical treatment has ceased. Second, the case illustrates the problems of adjustment that have to be overcome as nursing becomes divorced from the previously all-enveloping mantle of medical interpretation. The case examines the care delivered to Mrs Taylor (referred to earlier in Chapters 3 and 5), as she moves towards death. The narrative focuses on the period after the critical exchange between Mr Taylor and the senior registrar involved in her care, which was recounted in Chapter 5. A clear decision has been taken not to add anything to her treatment, and tentative preparations are in progress to transfer her to a ward so that the intensive care bed can be used for another patient.

Negotiating the meaning of technology in 'nursing care only'

The day after the interview between Mr Taylor and the senior registrar, I arrive on the unit to hear the nurses discussing what has been written by the medical staff in Mrs Taylor's notes and in the relatives' information sheet. They seem concerned that very little has actually been written down, and that they have to rely on a verbal account of the previous day's events. In the conversation that I have with Nurse J immediately after the bedside handover, she gives a clear account of her opinions regarding the most appropriate way in which to nurse Mrs Taylor from this point on, and reveals her perceptions of those factors which she feels constrain the delivery of such care:

> *07:00 – I arrived slightly late this morning, but heard the last part of the handover Nurse A to Nurse J. They are discussing what happened yesterday afternoon and reading the relatives' information sheet. J: 'They haven't written all of this in the notes.' (i.e. not for mini-trache, not for re-intubation, to the ward to 'let nature take its course'). J: 'It leaves us in the lurch when it's not written down in here.' – pointing to the red file.*

> *After A has gone, J tells me that the doctors are in theatres with a 'case': – 'So, she's on 70 per cent oxygen . . . I think it's awful. Why don't they give her a smidge of diamorphine, turn the oxygen down and just let her go. I think people are scared, you know, they just want to do the "right thing" and they get fazed by all of this (she gestures her hand in a sweeping motion around the unit). Do you know they (on the night shift) put an oral airway down and tried to suction her? "We didn't get anything up." Didn't get anything up! (She grumbles derisively) Why did they do it? She's not going to recover. Consultant A was only saying the other day: if it wasn't for these damned new fancy ventilators, she would have been taken off a lot sooner, put on facial cpap, we would have seen her struggling and a decision would have been easier. As it is, they messed about with cpap and asb [ventilatory modes], for ages. Mind you, he had said that no asb was to be given, but he didn't write it, and then someone else comes along and says: "Oh, her gases are crap, let's give her some asb!" The other thing is, if she was on a ward, she would've just gone to sleep and they would've found her dead – we just don't let that happen up here.'*

> *(Mrs Taylor appears to be unconscious, and she looks to me as if she is about to have a respiratory arrest.)*

> (From the field notes)

For J, the lack of a detailed written account by the medical staff leaves a vacuum of uncertainty around Mrs Taylor. She implies that her nursing care is contingent on a clarification (via documentation) of the intentions and role of the medical staff in the management of Mrs Taylor. She goes on further to describe how the availability of new techniques of ventilatory support have obscured and lengthened the process of recognizing that Mrs Taylor is approaching death. Further, she implies that the 'technical' environment engendered by the use of such equipment has encouraged the persistence of a particular style of nursing (characterized by the use of invasive suctioning techniques) even though it has been acknowledged that death is imminent.

Shortly after this exchange with J, the new duty consultant arrives to review the patients. The curtains are around Mrs Taylor's bed, because J and the support worker are washing her. The consultant listens to an account of the previous day's events given by the senior registrar, and then discusses with her the planned transfer to a surgical ward. At this point the curtains are drawn back from around the bed, and the discussion comes to a sudden stop; the appearance of Mrs Taylor (who is so obviously near death) arresting further conversation. Consultant B says slowly and in an embarrassed tone:

> 'Oh, . . . I think we may be keeping her here for a while – I think it would be inappropriate to move her – we have another bed don't we?'
> (From the field notes, day 18)

At this point J asks him about the exact details of Mrs Taylor's management. Consultant B seems keen to move to the next patient and tells her that the senior registrar will decide about these. The senior registrar goes through Mrs Taylor's prescription chart and 'crosses off' (discontinues the prescription) the few remaining drugs, and then instructs J to wait until Mrs Taylor's family have arrived but to then reduce the oxygen being delivered to her from 70 per cent to 35 per cent. From this moment there is no further medical involvement with Mrs Taylor; her management is left entirely to the nursing staff. The next extract from the field notes concerns the difference in interpretation, and obscured conflict, between nurses J and F, (the nurse who takes over from J), about what constituted 'nursing care' for Mrs Taylor.

> *13:00 – Nurse J hands over to Nurse F. They discuss whether or not she needs diamorphine. J says she is not sure; F wants to wait until the ward round and let the doctors decide: 'She looks asleep to me.' They talk about suction. F: 'Well, you can't let her drown, can you?' J: 'I don't think she needs it and I haven't given her any, I think she ought to be left in peace.' J goes on to explain to F that the SR has left instructions to reduce the oxygen from 70 per cent to 35 per cent, but not until the family is present (in case death is precipitated).*
>
> *13:45–14:15 – F sits at the end of the bed talking to another nurse. At 14:15, he gets up and looks at Mrs Taylor, he suctions her, using an airway and catheter. Mrs Taylor goes red in the face and retches. (J who is still on the unit sees this and says to me: 'I just wouldn't do that').*

14:30: Mr Taylor and his sister-in-law arrive. Mr Taylor kisses his wife; she does not manage to respond at all. They sit down several feet away from the bedside, both look distressed. Mr Taylor sits with his hands in his lap and his head bent; his sister-in-law sits next to him and stares at the monitor. F comes over to J who is at the central station near me, he says: 'Shall I turn the oxygen down now then? Why not put her on air – I don't go along with this half-way thing.' J whispers to him, I cannot hear what is being said. He returns to the bed and I see him reduce the oxygen. He says nothing to the family. He then starts to 'tidy up': moving monitoring equipment, disconnecting wires, and taking away pressure bags. I feel that he is 'preparing the way for death' but in a very instrumental and obvious way: no more need for checking the blood pressure or the oxygen saturation. F keeps himself busy like this – he smiles at Mr Taylor and the sister-in-law but does not stop to talk to them, they in their turn watch him while he works. F leaves the oxygen tubing attached to Mrs Taylor's face mask to drag under the bed – this has the effect of lifting the mask up so that it no longer covers her mouth or nose, but instead is over her eyes. Eventually, when neither he nor her family adjust it, J goes across and fixes the mask close to her face once more – she tucks the tubing under the pillow to stop it pulling again. Mrs Taylor is becoming grey, her breathing continues but she struggles for every breath. Death is imminent. F continues to tidy up and disappears with the equipment. The SR and the Consultant come round to Mrs Taylor's bed on the ward round, they have been with the newly admitted patient for the last 30 minutes. They stop at Mrs Taylor's bed and the SR says in a low voice: 'There's nothing to add here.' She shakes her head and points at the next bed. They move away and do not speak to Mr Taylor or his sister-in-law.

At 15:00 J prepares to go home. She goes across to Mr Taylor and his sister-in-law and squats down and speaks to them. She holds their hands in hers briefly. I leave shortly afterwards [I judge that it would be inappropriate to stay], and I also go over and speak to them, saying how sorry I am. They reply: 'Yes, but she looks peaceful, that's all we can hope for – thank-you for your attention.' We shake hands several times and I leave.

(From the field notes, day 18)

We see here a particularly stark (and possibly unusually divergent) example of widely differing views of 'nursing' in intensive care. Nurse J has to hand over to Nurse F and defers to his seniority of grade by not intervening overtly in Mrs Taylor's care from the point of the handover. Nurse F seems to attempt to confer with Nurse J and reach some sort of level of common ground. For instance, they discuss briefly whether or not Mrs Taylor needs diamorphine, and give their respective opinions about the use of suction. However, F takes an instrumental approach to Mrs Taylor, which is quite at odds with the more expressive approach of J. J sits at a distance, in apparent discomfort, while F busies himself with the equipment surrounding Mrs Taylor. He appears not to realize when Mrs Taylor's oxygen tubing becomes dislodged. J covertly adjusts the latter and expresses her unhappiness to me at F's actions in using suction on Mrs Taylor. J eventually leaves, but attempts to give some comfort to Mr Taylor and his sister-in-law before she does so. F, in contrast, concentrates his attentions on tidying away the various unnecessary pieces of monitoring equipment around Mrs Taylor.

Nurse F's concern with the equipment surrounding Mrs Taylor has the effect of placing a distance between him and her imminent death. He carries out his tasks in a 'day-to-day' fashion, as if nothing untoward is taking place. Mrs Taylor's dying, for F, seems incidental to his focus of work: the perpetuation of clinical competence and order with technology as the central feature. J's stance towards the technology surrounding Mrs Taylor is more critical, and her comments about its use in Mrs Taylor's treatment reveal an entirely different understanding of the relationship between nursing and technology to that conveyed by F. For J, technology simultaneously obscures the process of dying and obstructs the delivery of nursing care based on 'ordinary' notions of peaceful death.

Summary and discussion

An understanding of nursing work during dying must be rooted in detailed descriptions of what nurses actually do and feel in the particular situations in which they care for their patients (Bowden 1997: 105). As Benner *et al.* (1996) have argued, it is through such descriptions that common elements of nursing work may be identified and those aspects of nursing that are so difficult to articulate may be given voice.

This chapter has tried to 'give voice' to the complexity and sheer paradoxicality that attends the delivery of nursing care to dying people in intensive care. I have used the twin concepts of 'emotional work' and 'bodily work' showing how, far from nurses using bodily care as an escape from the demands of emotional engagement, in this environment it is an integral part of their emotional engagement not only with dying persons themselves but also with their companions. It is through these twin activities that nurses create 'whole person work' and invest the process of dying with meaning, purpose and intimacy. For some nurses, the compulsion to reproduce the subjectivity or 'personhood' of their patient is experienced as intensely painful. The case examples of Richard Morgan and Mr Randall, where we witnessed the recollections of two relatively inexperienced nurses, have given an insight into the depth of feelings that can be engendered by the demands that nursing ideology currently imposes.

Part of the problem faced by nurses in fashioning their work according to the predominant ideological strands of 'caring' and 'knowing the patient' within nursing, is that their work remains contingent on factors that are largely outside of their control. In the discussion of the problems experienced by nurses during the management of the nursing care of patients whose dying is characterized by divergence between the trajectories of 'technical' and 'bodily' death, we have seen how medical-technical imperatives, which are predicated on the separation of body and person, remain centrally placed. These imperatives operate effectively to exclude alternative perspectives on the situation of the dying person. Overarching this, as we saw in Chapter 6, is the tangled business of medical-technical rationalization with which doctors must engage in order to justify 'letting die'. In the intensive care situation any withdrawal of treatment may lead very quickly, perhaps almost precipitously, to death. Herein lies the problem of delayed dying that nurses experience as particularly distressing, and which challenges their notions of 'good nursing' so fundamentally. It is ironic to note, as Reiser (1992: 390, citing Hilberman 1975) observes in his citation of a physician's account of intensive care history, how important the predominantly nursing skills of 'intuition, experience and subliminal perception' were regarded by physicians in the early development of intensive care before mechanical means of monitoring patients' conditions had been developed. It seems that the development of highly technological means of 'reading' the patient, and the concomitant ethical problems that flow from greater technological surveillance, have contrived to force physicians largely to abandon this earlier stance and act instead, as we saw in the previous chapter, to bolster the legitimacy of 'technical dying' over and above 'bodily dying'.

What this chapter demonstrates most clearly is the extent to which nurses' understanding of 'good nursing' is entwined with notions of respect for personhood, bodily care and emotional investment. These are core elements of nursing that are embedded deeply in a wider socio-cultural understanding of the profession. And yet, as Bowden (1997) points out, it remains the case that 'caring', the concept that best describes the collision of these notions, is, and has been, systematically devalued by the societies and organizations to which nurses belong. As early as 1967, Quint (1967), latterly Quint-Benoliel (1977), highlighted the low status afforded to the 'caring' aspect of nursing, and the negative impact of this on the physical and psychological care of dying people. Quint-Benoliel highlighted the successful separation of such 'sex linked and interstitial tasks' (1977: 126) constituting the care of dying people, by a society that no longer embraced such intimate knowledge. She charted, in a detailed way, the problematic, paradoxical, and powerless situation of nurses within the medicalized

environment of the hospital. She described how nurses must atten
intimate 'care' needs of dying patients within a depersonalized environ...
predicated on the denial of death and the procuration of 'cure'. Drawing
on the work of Menzies (1970), who suggested that nursing services within
hospitals developed particular kinds of social 'systems' to protect nurses
from the psychological pressures induced by the demands of caring work,
Quint-Benoliel argued that nurses' location on the cure-care continuum
was a major contributor to their experiences of disabling distress and anxiety.

For most nurses the obligation, indeed the *compulsion*, to care is accompanied by an inability to express the value of care in a currency that others
understand, and a lack of authority to influence the environment in which
caring activities take place. It is during dying that these tensions become
highly visible and when nurses struggle most to enact that which has long
been a quintessential part of their role.

Note

1 The term 'nursing care only' has been drawn from my own nursing experience:
it is not something that has been deconstructed in the relevant literature, but is
referred to as 'full nursing care' in Mackay (1993: 147). It became a particular
issue in this research as a result of a field note taken in case 6 Eastern, when I
noted that the consultant had written 'for nursing care only' in the medical notes.

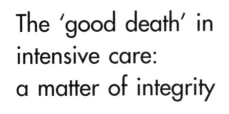

8 The 'good death' in intensive care: a matter of integrity

Professional discourse about 'good' death has become a central reference point for wider ideas about a 'natural' time and 'way' of dying. It is characterized predominantly by reference to ideas about the facilitation of awareness of dying, development of conscious self-identity, and social and psychological preparation for death. However, the application of these ideas to deaths occurring in intensive care is, at first sight, problematic. When it occurs, death in intensive care is almost always marked by the extreme vulnerability and bodily dependence of the dying person and by an apparent lack or impairment of their awareness of 'self'. This is a result of unconsciousness due in part to the severity of their underlying biological state, and in part to the induction of an 'artificial' state by sedative and analgesic drugs administered to relieve the inevitable pain of illness and the discomfort caused by intensive care treatments. It seems, then, that this is the image of death 'dissected' (Ariès 1976) from its connection with the natural world and thrown into an arena where the processes of bodily dying are delayed, concealed and subverted; and resignation and awareness of a predictable order of natural events is replaced by a fragile hope for recovery, and the uncertainty and risk of an unpredictable chaos of technologically determined events. Most critically, the exercise of choice, control and self-determination by the dying person, so central to the dominant ideologies of good death, is impossible.

In spite of these features of death in intensive care, opportunities to negotiate and orchestrate 'good' deaths do arise. Where these were achieved during this study, they were marked by the sustenance of what can be conceptualized as a multi-faceted form of 'integrity'. The term implies an internally consistent, coherent state and is used usually to refer to 'conventional standards of morality, especially those of truth telling, honesty and fairness' (McFall 1987: 5). In the literature related to death and dying it has been used both to describe an 'ideal' relationship between dying people and their professional carers, and to delineate those elements that may contribute to a sense of personal or professional 'disintegration' during the process of dying (Saunders and Valente 1994; Miller and Brody 1995; de Raeve 1996). This chapter focuses on the recollections of death and near death narrated by patients' companions, using these to develop insight into the conditions in which 'disintegration' is prevented. In so doing some sense is gained of how meaning is ascribed creatively, through story telling, to death-related experiences long after the events to which they refer took place.

At an early stage of data analysis, particular themes were noted within companions' recollections of patients' deaths or near deaths. These were concerned with bodily care and appearance, trust, emotional exchange, and the reproduction of meaningful personhood. As these were applied to a further analysis of the data, a re-working of the concept of 'integrity' gradually emerged, in which several interrelated elements were identified:

- maintenance of the integrity of the 'natural order'
- maintenance of the integrity of the dying individual's personhood
- maintenance of trust between healthcare staff and patients' companions.

Identification of these core elements allowed a 'good death' in intensive care to be outlined as that in which a navigation of technology achieves death at an expected and appropriate time and place; peacefulness and painlessness are engendered; and companions are present. Furthermore, in 'good deaths' the individuality of the dying person is protected by bodily care and by an expressed respect for his or her social being, meaning and place within the family. Such deaths are also characterized by the development of a trusting and reciprocal relationship between the companions of the dying individual and the healthcare 'experts' who mediate between them. This trust and reciprocity is marked by an exchange of intimacy and emotion, which, although temporary, seems to have long-lasting effects on the perception and recollections of companions.

This chapter examines each of these elements in turn. To begin, perceptions of the relationship between medical technology and 'natural death' will be examined, focusing on ideas companions expressed about the influence of technology on serious illness and death. Attention then turns to accounts of the meaning and value of the reproduction of personhood by means of bodily care, before concluding with an examination of the importance to companions of creating close, trusting relationships with healthcare staff.

Integrity of the 'natural order'

First we turn to the 'fusion and confusion' (Hockey 1996: 14) of medical technology and 'nature' that surrounds death in intensive care and to ideas

Table 8.1   Categories of expectation and outcome

Companions' expectation	Resulting outcome	Related cases (Eastern; Western)
1 Probable death	life	case 5E; cases 3,6W
2 Probable death	death	cases 1,2,6,8E; cases 1,2W
3 Probable life	death	cases 3,4,7E; cases 4,5W

about how the integrity of the 'natural order' of death are represented by companions. In particular, it shows how their experiences are fashioned by their expectations concerning the success or failure of medical technology: the fulfillment of these expectations is revealed as a critical constituent of the 'natural' and the natural order of events.

The case studies completed during the research on which this book is based can be categorized according to the particular expectations about death that were expressed by the companions of each patient. Three broad patterns of expectation and related outcome can be identified (the term probable has been used to emphasize the presence of uncertainty in each of the groups).[1,2] These are shown in Table 8.1.

Analysis of the data available about the cases that fell within each of these three categories revealed the central role of expectation in the formulation of ideas about technology and its link to 'natural' or 'unnatural' deaths. In the first category, where death was seen as the most likely outcome of a companion's illness, and yet life resulted, some markedly paradoxical perceptions were expressed regarding the relationship between technology, death and the natural order of events. Technology was seen as something essentially mysterious, unpredictable and miraculous: its application was seen as a subversion of events *even* in the two cases where the aversion of death was greeted with extreme relief and joy. In the second pattern, where death was expected and occurred, an emphasis was placed on the role of technology in achieving the 'ideal' natural order with which death should be attended. Here death occurred at an appropriate, 'natural' time in which technical dying was confirmed *before* bodily death took place, and where staff and companions could enact particular, expected roles. These roles were characterized by acceptance of death and validation of the curative orientation of intensive care. In the third pattern, where death occurred unexpectedly, the failure of technology to deliver the recovery that had been expected was linked to an interruption of the natural order of events and to the wider risks and failures of an unpredictable and unsafe healthcare system.

One case representing each of the three patterns will be presented here. In each of these cases the designated next of kin completed a follow-up interview, during which we talked about their expectations and feelings while their companion was ill and after their death or recovery.

Expected death – life as the outcome: the subversion of 'natural death'

> Mr Cook was a 54-year-old man admitted to intensive care with a severe pneumonia and septicaemia. He was in intensive care for 12 days and eventually recovered enough to be transferred to a ward. From there he was discharged home. He had a long history of chronic physical and mental illness. His companion was his estranged wife, who, although living apart from him, had continued to assume responsibility for his day-to-day care.

Mr Cook's long history of illness and suffering, which was described by his wife, appeared to have had a particular influence on her perceptions of the role of technology in his care. In my interpretation she viewed her husband's unexpected recovery as a *failure* of technology rather than a success. This was because she felt that what had occurred had intervened in the *natural* course of his dying. For her, this intervention meant that she and her children had not only to endure a further period of extreme practical difficulty as they struggled to care for Mr Cook, but also to give care in the almost certain knowledge that, eventually, all the distressing feelings associated with his imminent death would be re-experienced.

In her follow-up interview five months later, Mrs Cook communicated a sense of confusion and anger about the subversion of what she had perceived to be the natural, expected course of events by technological innovation. A central part of her account concerns her perception of intensive therapy as disconnected both from the wider context of her husband's life and from the prolonged anxiety experienced during the years in which she had struggled to care for him and in which she had witnessed the gradual decline in his mental and physical health. She went on to describe how, when he was finally admitted to hospital having been found in a collapsed state, she felt relieved that he was 'in the right hands' and that 'someone else was in charge'. His confused and critically ill condition on the general ward at this time confirmed her suspicion that he would almost certainly die, but at this point he is transferred to intensive care and there is an immediate improvement in his state. This leaves her feeling profoundly uncertain as to what the eventual outcome is likely to be:

R: I'd had desperate stress about him since the summer . . . I didn't know what to think. I was relieved that someone was in charge, that he was in the right hands . . . Then, having been not lucid at all on the wards, the very first day on intensive care he had a very lucid conversation with his children, the clearest he'd had in months. That was very, very weird you know – having got ready for him dying and then to see how lucid he was, and how much he had come round; it was very strange.

JS: How did that leave you feeling?

R: Very messed around actually -- I mean it *was* wonderful that he got better and responded; people do get better, but a lot of people don't survive, and that prolonging of that period is very hard on relatives because you sort of gear yourself up to accepting it and then you are sort of kept in limbo I think -- I just felt, we all felt, well, we've just got all this to go through again soon. We were just sort of waiting for it to all start again.

JS: Did you feel as if you had any control over what was being done to him?

R: Um -- not really. I was *told* what the situation was while he was in intensive care, and how ill he was and everything. Before he came round, I did tell the nurses – it was a terrible thing to say really – but I said: 'all this money is being poured into him to keep him alive and he'll just start up again at home'; and the next thing I knew he was down on the ward and they had said that they wouldn't ventilate him again. I thought that was my fault (laughs) I didn't think they'd take me seriously!

(From follow-up interview)

It is clear here that Mrs Cook portrays herself as preparing for, and accepting, a death which does not occur, and which is instead merely delayed: she foresees her suffering, and that of her husband and children, as being prolonged rather than alleviated by the course of events. Her perception that the nurses acted on her communication to them of her feelings about the appropriateness of the high technology treatments is coupled with a belief that she had no real control over events even though she was given information relating to the seriousness of his condition. These impressions are confirmed later in the interview when she describes how she felt 'fragile' and 'almost bereaved' during the initial period of Mr Cook's admission:

We weren't expecting him to pull through and we weren't given much indication that he would pull through, so I don't know, for two nights in particular on the wards, it was just like waiting for him to die. At first I thought when he was on intensive care . . . well, really, I didn't know what to think. I hadn't a clue what was happening, I hadn't a clue. As I say, at first, I thought, I was impressed by what they could do, but then I thought, well, this is only prolonging how long it takes him to die. I started to question it actually. I felt it was prolonging it, spinning it out, I thought, well, six years ago this all wouldn't have

been here and is it a good thing or not? It was an extra period of limbo
-- it's only natural getting upset and grieving, but it spins it out.

(From follow-up interview)

She goes on to describe intensive care, and hospital care in general, as
'another world' fundamentally unrelated to the realities with which she was
engaged on a day-to-day basis and unresponsive to either her needs or
those of her husband. It is within the context of this account of the unre-
sponsiveness and irrelevance of healthcare technology that Mrs Cook's
perceptions regarding her husband's survival can be understood. In effect,
his 'salvation' by the application of medical science is interpreted as a
bizarre subversion, or twist, of the 'natural' course of a chronic illness that
had almost run its full extent. The sudden application of medical technology at a time when her husband was 'nearly dead' and after a period of
time in which she had struggled, apparently with little support, to give
attention to his most basic human needs, is represented as an illogical and
cruel interruption of the natural sequence of events in which death would
have followed, bringing with it a release from suffering, anxiety and ardu-
ous caring.

This case perhaps fits the classic model of an 'unnatural' event in the midst
of high technology intervention in which the application of technology is
essentially out of step with ordinary perceptions of the dying trajectory
and in which the processes of dying are thwarted, hidden and thrown off
course in ways which are essentially inaccessible to lay understandings,
knowledge or control. The next example, however, focuses on a contrasting perception of death as timely, compassionate and humanized in spite of
its occurrence within a similarly highly technical setting.

Probable death – death as the outcome: the role of technology in achieving an 'ideal' death

> This section concerns the case of Mrs Richards, a 73-year-old woman
> admitted to intensive care with a diagnosis of pneumonia and septicaemia.
> Mrs Richards died after a withdrawal of cardiovascular drug support, three
> days after her admission to intensive care.

We were introduced to Mrs Richards' situation in Chapter 3. The focus
here concerns several key characteristics of the 'technologically controlled'
death of Mrs Richards and their relationship to the negotiation of the
natural order that took place during and after her death. The characteristics of technological control engendered the conditions in which the

trajectory of death was adjusted to ensure four factors. First, that the process of dying was neither too prolonged nor too precipitate. Second, that 'technical death' could be aligned to 'bodily death' thereby legitimating the medical control of events and ensuring that death only occurred once all avenues of possible treatment were exhausted. Third, that Mrs Richards' awareness of dying was suppressed and her family's acceptance of death facilitated. Lastly, technological control engendered an environment in which the family was able to witness a gradual, quiet and dignified event. Below is an extract from the field notes taken shortly before Mrs Richards' death, which reveals clearly the features of technological control that surrounded it. Mrs Richards' daughters are at her bedside and the cardiovascular drug support she is receiving is about to be withdrawn:

Staff Nurse B comes out of the room to allow the sisters to be on their own with their mother. She tells me that they will wait until the third sister arrives before the drugs are stopped. I ask whether they will be reduced gradually or just turned off. B tells me: 'I think they will just be turned off'. The registrar who is listening to our conversation says: 'Sometimes its better just to turn everything off and then the family can see that the patient was only being kept alive artificially – they understand when they die quickly that there was no chance of survival.' B is more cautious than this: 'I think that sometimes they need it to be slower, to get used to the idea, and anyway sometimes some people seem to rally temporarily when all the drugs are switched off.'

13:30 B goes back to the bedside and prepares to hand over to Staff Nurse C for the start of the late shift.

14:30: The third sister has arrived. Staff Nurse B comes out of the room leaving Nurse C with the three sisters and Mrs Richards. B looks worried: 'Where's Dr Y, I want to know what to turn off and in what order.' She dashes off to find Dr Y, saying: 'They're all here now and I don't want a mess made of it.'

15:00 Dr Y goes into the room with Nurse B. He comes out shortly afterwards and tells me that they have turned off the inotropes, left the sedation and turned the oxygen down from 100 per cent to 30 per cent.

The three daughters are in the room with Nurse C. The door is shut and the blind pulled. At 16:00 C comes out for a short break and a cup of tea. Two of the sisters come out as well, and they go to sit in the curtained off relatives' room. Susan is left in her mother's room on her own. I decide that it is time for me to leave and ask C tentatively whether I may go and say goodbye to Susan. C agrees to my request and I go into the room quietly. Mrs Richards is obviously near death; Susan is holding her hand. I speak to her, telling her that I am leaving and that I will be thinking of her and her sisters. She says goodbye to me and then: 'This is what we want – like this.'

(From field notes)

During the follow-up interview that I was able to complete with Susan four months later, she gave some insight into the meaning for her of this technological management of her mother's death. She recalled first her relief that she could 'hand over' responsibility for the care of her mother to the intensive care staff:

I didn't have to worry about trying to look after her needs myself. Downstairs, they were good, but couldn't be there all the time -- I was worried all the time, you know in case she took her oxygen mask off or something. Up there that responsibility was gone, I could hand that over to the staff (who) were simply more competent and more used to dealing with people in that situation ...

(From follow-up interview)

She goes on to recall how she could 'see' that her mother was not going to recover, and indicated that having time to incorporate this view with the account given to her by the medical staff allowed her to accept the inevitability of death. She re-presents the version of events given to her by the senior registrar and in so doing gives an almost instrumental account of her mother's death. We are left with an impression of a death that was 'good' precisely because it happened in such a controlled and technological environment:

I think very quickly after she'd been admitted to intensive care, we realized and the doctors were perfectly honest with us, that it was, the odds were against her getting better and at that stage when we realized she was deteriorating so fast, our attitude was sort of to say to the doctors, you know: 'At your convenience withdraw drug support from her' because that was purely what was keeping her alive -- we were warned when she was admitted that she was -- one of the sickest patients there, so I realized at that stage, or at least had it confirmed, how ill she was. I think the seeds were sown then that: 'No, she's not going to get any better.' Her kidneys had failed; they'd tried various methods of physical and drug induced [treatment] to kick start her but it was only a matter of making a difference for a matter of hours ... it was just a matter that once we realized that she wasn't going to get better then you know, fine, let's get on with it.

(From follow-up interview)

Susan's account of the actual moment of death reveals how important the timing of that event was: in the extract below we witness a managed, 'technological' death, in which the very application of technology allows for a peaceful scene characterized by family proximity, dignity and respect for Mrs Richards as an individual:

> *JS*: Did you feel that they handled the way in which she died as you wanted it?
>
> *R*: Yes, yes, for instance my other sister was coming over from [town] and they said: 'We've started withdrawing drug support, but if we think she's going to fade before your sister comes then we'll put something back in to keep her going' and as it got very close to the end they turned off the monitors and it was only when the nurse was sort of holding the pulse they then said 'It was over' which was nice not to see because obviously she was on a ventilator so even after she'd gone her chest was still breathing in effect. Yes I've nothing but praise for the way she was treated even to the fact that things have been run down and we knew it was only a matter of minutes, they still washed her face and wiped the gunk out of her mouth and that. To give her as much dignity and respect, they did [for] whatever feelings or sensations she still had, she was being treated the best she could -- all along when they were treating her I mean especially since she was in intensive care she was never conscious so it wasn't somebody they knew, she was continually being treated as an individual rather than something on a production line.
>
> *JS*: Did you expect that before you went in or did you not know what to expect?
>
> *R*: I wasn't quite sure how much they would treat her as an individual and I found that very nice.
>
> (From follow-up interview)

Susan's account of her mother's death shows how it was possible for her to preserve some sense of the rightful place and natural sequence of events: death occurred only after it had become clear that such an outcome was inevitable and after all treatment options were exhausted. The ability to adjust the timing of death and its occurrence within a controlled environment in which the very moment of death was disguised, were, for Susan, important and meaningful features. They ensured that she could, together with her sisters, attend the final moments of her mother's life, and witness a quiet, dignified, and gradual event. Thus, in spite of the sudden onset of her mother's illness and the extreme technological interventions instituted, the actual moment of death is recollected as timely, and its management portrayed as essentially compassionate and humanized rather than, as might be expected by an outside observer, the technological invasion of the body being *deterministic* of dehumanized death.

The two cases examined so far show how the application of human agency via medical technology may be represented as either supportive or unsupportive of 'natural' death. We can see that this representation depends on the type of expectations held concerning the illness trajectories and also on the emergence within companions of some sense of involvement in, and understanding of, the events taking place during the process of dying. The example chosen to represent the next pattern, in which expectation does not match outcome, focuses more closely on the importance to respondents of 'making sense' of the relationship between illness, death, medicine and medical technology. We see that where professional explanations about medicine, illness and technology do not 'fit' with ordinary understandings or knowledge, then the perception of, or construction of 'natural' death becomes impossible to sustain.

Probable life – death as the outcome: the betrayal of faith in medical technology

> Mrs Stafford was a 71-year-old woman, who was admitted to intensive care in Western hospital 15 days after undergoing elective surgery for resection of carcinoma of the bowel. Mrs Stafford had a husband (John) and a daughter (Pat). Mrs Stafford's initial post-operative recovery was uneventful, but she gradually developed signs of dehydration, renal impairment, pneumonia, and septicaemia, eventually becoming critically ill with respiratory failure and depressed consciousness. She was transferred initially from a surgical ward to the high dependency unit, but was transferred to the adjoining intensive care unit following a further acute deterioration in her condition. She recovered enough to be discharged from intensive care on day eight. Six days after her transfer from intensive care Mrs Stafford suffered a further acute deterioration in her condition, culminating in a cardio-respiratory arrest. Following an unsuccessful resuscitation attempt she died, 27 days post-operatively.

A follow-up interview was completed with John and Pat, five months after Mrs Stafford's death. During the course of the interview (in which Pat was the main spokesperson) they described vividly the events leading up to Mrs Stafford's illness and portrayed her eventual death as an inexplicable betrayal of their faith in medical expertise and technology. This interview appeared (in my interpretation) to be an attempt by the respondents to 'make sense' of death by the production of a consensual account of deeply distressing experiences.

Pat recalled how, shortly after her mother had been diagnosed as suffering from cancer, they had received reassurances from both the general practitioner and from the consultant surgeon at the hospital about the high likelihood of survival following the planned surgery. This confidence is re-affirmed immediately after the operation, when Pat goes to visit her mother and finds her sitting up in bed, looking comparatively well:

Pat: We went on the Monday night.

John: She was talking.

Pat: Yes, she kept going to sleep, but, as she was sat up, her stomach – it had been out here – and as they sat her up, because of her breathing, it had gone! It was just, my mum was amazed herself, she just kept pointing to her stomach, she just couldn't believe where her stomach had gone, and you know, she was dozing off, but she looked really 100 per cent, she looked the best she'd looked for years and years, she looked really fit.

(From follow-up interview)

Pat goes on to recall her realization several days later that her mother was becoming ill with a high temperature and confusion. She describes how, having been summoned urgently to the hospital, she finds herself at the forefront of efforts to galvanize the healthcare staff into the urgent activity she feels they should be taking to save her mother. Furthermore, the explanations she receives about the cause of her mother's deterioration confuse her since they do not 'fit' with her understanding of medical science. It is at this point that the environment surrounding her mother becomes interpreted as unsafe, unpredictable and out of keeping with the earlier confident expectation of the trajectory of recovery. In the extract below, Pat describes the appearance of her mother shortly before her transfer to the high dependency unit:

Pat: She just didn't know anything and she were rambling, and all spit were [*sic*] down here. It was just so poor, that ward was so poor really. They'd moved my mum closer to the windows so they could look after her, but we couldn't believe it – she looked as though she was dying there and then. And anyway, we said, well, you've brought us here, what's going to be done now? They said: 'We're waiting for the Doctor', and all the time we seemed to be saying: 'I want', but if we didn't, nothing seemed to happen. We said: 'Look, can you get someone to see to mum because she's not right – look at her, she's so poorly.' -- Anyway Doctor came and he said: 'Right, we're going to take her up to high dependency'.

JS: Did you know what was the matter with her?

Pat: We never knew what was the matter with her. All they kept saying was that mum had got a bug in the blood, that's all they kept saying, a bug in the blood. Well, for someone who is not medical, you can get rid of bugs with tablets, so as far as we were concerned there was nothing wrong with her, because a bug in the blood, what's a bug in the blood?

John: They can cure it.

Pat: That's it. Anyway, she went up to high dependency and by this time she was completely out of it; she'd just slipped into a coma . . . The doctor said to us, 'I've got to tell you, Mrs Stafford isn't going to pull through'. And we just turned round and said: 'You what?' For someone to turn round and say that after she had been so perfectly well after such a big operation -- just didn't seem to sink in -- and you can imagine it we were all crying, we were just devastated -- it was just a horrible experience, I don't ever want to experience anything like it ever again.

(From follow-up interview)

At this point Mrs Stafford is moved into intensive care and starts to make a recovery. Pat recalls how she begins to regain some sense of confidence in her mother's treatment and hopes for an eventual recovery. However, these hopes are unfulfilled. Her mother dies suddenly, without her family being present, a few days after her transfer from intensive care. Pat describes her feeling that with the move from intensive care to the ward, they had been moved from 'rich to poor' (interview data), and both she and her father voice their firm belief that if Mrs Stafford had stayed in intensive care she would have survived:

John: What I can't understand is this, they knew there was something wrong that night – why didn't they take her back into the intensive care? I'm sure if she'd been taken back up there -- (he shakes his head sadly).

Pat: It could turn nasty, Mum was starting to do perfectly well and from doing that to and then to die; its absolutely heartbreaking . . .

John: 'Cause she had gone through all that and then . . .

Pat: She died.

John: Yeah.

JS: You seem to be saying that you have been left not understanding why?

John: Oh, I think so. They kept taking blood tests and this and that and the other, and no one said anything, did they?

Pat: When he said, Dr X, that your Mum's got brain damage, we don't know why she'd got brain damage. We don't know why. We don't know all the way. I mean, this might sound gory, but to me, it's like my mum's been murdered. I know it's awful to say it, but that's how I feel . . . to have someone so healthy after the operation and in theory, it was the operation that was the problem -- well, you just think 100 per cent all the time don't you? But unfortunately it wasn't to be. All I know is that it was septicaemia, and that's poison of the blood. But you can get rid of a poison can't you?

(From follow-up interview)

This extreme description of death as 'murder' can be seen as representing the archetypal, 'unnatural' death. As in the example of Mrs Richards, the application of technology fails to secure survival, but the circumstances in which death occurs are very different. Pat and John are unable to locate the death within their idea of the boundaries of medical science: it seems inconceivable to them that an apparently routine 'bug in the blood' could have so cruelly interrupted the predicted course of their mother/wife's post-operative recovery. Moreover, in their interpretation, the use of technology was inconsistent, unreliable and unable to pre-empt signs of her sudden demise. This threatens a worldview in which medicine is predictable, safe and fully able to apprehend the workings of the body. Unlike Mrs Richards's daughter Susan, who could recall how death occurred in a controlled environment in which all avenues of treatment had been exhausted, Pat and John communicate a sense of extreme suspicion regarding the circumstances surrounding death. For them, death occurs without warning and in uncontrolled circumstances: they cannot align the explanations that they have been given with their conception of what *should have been* the rightful, natural, logical course of events. They can only regard her death as a sign of the abject failure of medical surveillance and care.

Integrity of personhood

In the previous chapter, attention focused on the central role of bodily care in nursing work in intensive care. We saw how nursing care is constituted by an alignment of 'body work' with 'emotional work' and how this allows the reproduction of subjectivity within the bodies of ill and dying people. Below, attention will focus on the *meaning* of such bodily care for the close companions of the critically ill individuals. It will be shown that particular styles of bodily care and management are critical in the preservation of the individuality or 'person' of the ill individual for his or her companions. Reference has been made earlier in this chapter to the importance of bodily care in the recollections of Mrs Richards's daughter Susan, and in the previous chapter, some brief reference was made to the recollections of the wife and son of Mr Hart. They remembered that the close attention to the bodily appearance of Mr Hart confirmed his social worth, and was in keeping with their own intimate, family feelings for him. These recollections will be explored in more detail here and a comparison drawn between the account given by Mr Hart's son and wife and that given by Mrs Stafford's daughter. Taken together, the stories from the two families suggest that the recollections of the bodily care of dying people, and whether or not this was perceived as supportive of their individuality or 'person', are of central importance in the construction of accounts of death. Furthermore, it will be shown that interpretations of the meaning of bodily care depend on relationships of trust between companions and healthcare staff, and, as indicated earlier, on the ability of companions to locate the death within a coherent, predictable and *understandable* series of events.

To begin, we return to the case of Mrs Stafford introduced above, and focus on the way in which her daughter drew a comparison between the bodily management of her mother in intensive care and that delivered on the general wards. The former is seen as both *supportive* of Mrs Stafford's individuality and of the emotional needs of her husband and her daughter, Pat. The latter, in contrast, is seen as a *threat* both to Mrs Stafford's individuality and to the well-being of her family. A vivid description is provided in which the themes of bodily respect, bodily desecration and the preservation of the mother–daughter relationship predominate. Pat's account is revealing because she is able to describe times when her mother was fully unconscious, as well as those brief periods in which her mother was beginning to return to a more awake, although confused, state.

Bodily management as a threat to personhood

A repeated theme in Pat's interview was the importance to her of her mother's bodily care and appearance. For Pat, such care preserved her mother's dignity and was a mark of the overall quality of the care and treatment she was receiving. Pat describes, for example, how she had asked the surgical ward staff if they could provide her mother with a bath. She interprets their partial refusal as a more general indicator of poor care:

> *She didn't have a bath -- I kept asking because she smelt terrible. They said: 'She's on the list for tomorrow.' I said: 'She needs one today!' I think she was neglected. If she had been up here none of it would ever have happened. I could see she was bad, my dad could see she was bad. I know the professionals know what's what, but she's my mother.*

> (From the field notes)

In her follow-up interview Pat contrasts the level of physical attention provided on the ward with that provided in intensive care, and gives some indication of what this meant to her:

> *Pat:* [in intensive care] they even had her sat up, out of bed! She had her hair done and she looked absolutely [great] . . . they really, really took a lot of time and considered your feelings. I mean there was a lady, called, er, Nurse X, and she talked to my mum like my mum would have talked back to her. She said: 'Come on now Mrs Stafford, get out of bloody bed!' and (laughing) My mum says: 'Bugger off, I don't want to get out of bed!' And as soon as we knew that she

was answering people like that, we knew that she were getting better. This nurse, she didn't put on any airs and graces. She said: 'Do your mum's hair, because it might make her feel better,' and it did. When she went down to the ward she looked like a million dollars didn't she?

John: Yes, yes.

(From follow-up interview)

In this account Pat recalls that seeing the nurses spending time with her mother gave her the sense that her own feelings, as well as those of her mother, were being considered. Further, she remembers the physical nursing care being given in a personal way, taking account of her mother's particular personality. Pat also gives the impression that, by participating in the care of her mother, she was able to reach some mutual level of understanding with the nurse over her mother's condition and, she implies, preserve her relationship with her mother:

> *Pat*: when we were there, intensive care, they used to say can you excuse us, or, we'll bring you some hot water and you can wash your mum, you know, and even down to little bits of when my mum was in a coma and she was on a ventilator and there was this stuff in her mouth. They used this suction thing, you've seen it haven't you? And that nurse, said: 'Take this and do your mum's mouth out and suck it out.' I was frightened to put it in but when I did, she moved her tongue out of the way, you know! Even down to that, it might be stupid, but I was helping to look after my own mum.
>
> *JS*: And was that important?
>
> *Pat*: Yes it were [*sic*]. I cleaned her stomach as well, and it was clean.

(From follow-up interview)

In Pat's subsequent account of her feelings of grief and regret over the death of her mother, she refers to her feeling that she was in some way 'let down' by a particular member of the intensive care staff with whom she had developed a trusting relationship. Further, she and her father describe how they developed an impression that the medical treatment Mrs Stafford was given subsequently was lacking:

> *Pat*: I was worried about going away to [city for the weekend] on the Friday, and X the staff nurse said: 'Don't worry, your mother will not leave this ward until I say that she is fit enough'. Unfortunately he went off sick and I just wonder, in the back of my mind, whether my mum would still be here now if he hadn't. Because they wouldn't have moved her out so quickly . . .
>
> *John*: I think they took her out too early -- if they'd kept her in a bit longer, I think she'd have come round -- What I can't understand is that when they took her back to that other ward, I knew something

was wrong with her again, and they knew as well -- they took her down for a scan didn't they?

Pat: It was like being back at square one again weren't it Dad [*sic*]?

(From follow-up interview)

It is this lack of understanding regarding her management that is later re-presented by Pat as a picture in which she imagines that her mother's body has been mutilated in some way. These impressions seem to be related to the particularly confusing and sudden circumstances (described earlier) in which death occurred and from which Pat and John were absent. Pat discloses that she had been convinced that her mother's legs had been somehow removed from her body, and that this image has been difficult to erase from her mind. The reason she gives for this image is the odd appearance of her mother's dead body under the sheet: she describes the body as having a huge distended stomach, so that the sheet fell sharply away from the middle of the bed and made it appear that the legs were missing. She relates this fear to the witnessing of all the physical interventions that her mother had to endure just before death and the evidence of which linger long after death:

Ten days after my mum died and she were in a coffin, she'd still got great big, bloody marks in her hands where they'd took blood off her. I couldn't understand this because she'd got this thing [intravenous cannula] in her neck, so why couldn't they use that. Eventually this doctor came in and I said: 'You're not taking no more out of her!' My mum's hand had swollen and it were like phlebitis, and I said; 'You can't stick that in my mum.' All the time I were hurting [*sic*]; I don't know if my mum were 'cause she were half and half asleep [*sic*], but she must have been.

(From follow-up interview)

This enduring interpretation of bodily management as indicative of bodily desecration is related to Pat's earlier accounts of medical treatment as unsafe, unpredictable and inconsistent, and to her lack of comprehension of the bodily processes that have caused death. Further, she and her father did not *predict* the occurrence of death. This is confirmed in their account of their memories of the hours before death, where they seem to negotiate between them in order to produce an 'accurate' shared account of the finest details of events during those hours (even involving me in the constructive attempt at one point). By reference to such small, everyday details they search in their recollections for signs of imminent death. The marked sadness and desolation at the end of their account seems to be related to the shock of an unexpected, and in their terms, inexplicable, event:

Pat: On the Saturday, as it were my birthday [*sic*], I went to see my mum. Took my dad up, dropped him off first, Dad sat with Mum, gave her a bit of rice pudding. You better tell her now because I don't know from this bit.

John: I took some rice pudding, put it in this basin and she had a bit of rice pudding. Then she says: 'I don't want no more.' So that were it. And then she says: 'Are you stopping tonight?'

Pat: Oh! Did she say that to you?

John: Yes. 'Are you stopping tonight.' I says: 'No. Why?' She says: 'I'm frightened.' I says: 'What have you got to be frightened of? There's all these people here!' And then she fell asleep.

Pat: Yeah.

John: Fast asleep.

Pat: Yes.

John: I stopped by her until . . .

Pat: Six o'clock.

John: Oh it were after that!

Pat: Because I came to collect you.

John: Aye. Aye.

Pat: But, I went to the hospital and it was my birthday that day and my dad had sent me a card, and I -- er, I went -- this was the last time I spoke to my mum -- I went up and I went to the side of the bed and I kept looking at her and I kept (miming touching her); and my dad kept going like this (miming touch) and she *used* to say; 'gerroff' (laughs) she didn't like to be covered up or to be touched, she would have thrown herself away; but she didn't do this. So, I thought then, this is not normal, to let me do this to her. My father was still sat there and then I says: 'Dad, come on, we're going home now.' As soon as my dad stood up, she woke up like that didn't she; her eyes were wide open! And er, I said: 'You're something to wake up now!' I said: We're going off home because my dad's got a blonde coming.' And she says: 'Well, he won't keep her bloody waiting then had he?' (Laughter). And that was my mum. That was the good side of my mum. I said to her: 'You've not said happy birthday to me today.' She said: 'Happy birthday' and that were the last I spoke to her . . . I just, I couldn't tell you what went wrong at all. Although she were very poorly, she were very tired [*sic*]. They just 'phoned up on the Sunday morning at twenty past eight.

John: At nine o'clock.

Pat: And they said come, come up because your mum's very poorly . . .

John: And Dr X were there weren't he? Do you know Dr X?

JS: I've heard the name.

John: And they took us into this little room and they said: 'Your mum's got brain damage.' And she'd only had a scan two days before and it was alright. So we don't know.

(long pause)

Pat: (sighing) And that were it. It's just so bad. I can't think of what --
of what to say.

(From follow-up interview)

We turn now to examine a case in which bodily care and management are
construed as a *support* of 'person', even in the face of visible bodily deterioration during the process of dying.

The meaning of bodily care: a support to personhood

We return here to the case of Mr Hart, introduced in Chapters 5 and 7. Mr
Hart was a 74-year-old man admitted for treatment of a severe head injury.
It was acknowledged early in the nine-day course of his intensive care
treatment that Mr Hart would almost certainly die, and this prediction was
communicated to his wife and son by the healthcare staff. This crucial
difference in predictability between the trajectory of Mr Hart's death and
that of Mrs Stafford seems to influence the recollections of Mr Hart's
wife and son regarding the management of his body. In contrast to Mrs
Stafford's family, they are able to recollect how bodily management and
care was *supportive* of Mr Hart's personhood, even when he had been transferred from intensive care to a ward, and in circumstances in which the
withdrawal of intravenous fluids and naso-gastric feeding rendered a rapid
deterioration in his bodily appearance. This interpretation seemed to depend on their ability to sustain a sense of involvement in, and understanding of the events leading up to death. It is this sense of involvement and
understanding that is so lacking in the account proffered by Pat and John
Stafford.

The feelings of involvement and understanding possessed by Mr Hart's
son and wife seem to be related in part to previous experience. Thus
Mr Hart's son, Michael, is able to say how:

I think because of [x] we could see a lot of the information for
ourselves . . . we could understand the fact that once different tubes
and bags were taken away it wasn't, in my dad's case, a sign that he
were getting better. It were a sign that they were closing down as such,
and doing it in the nicest way possible . . . being able to understand the
technology is a great thing I think, and it certainly helps.

(From follow-up interview)

Mr Hart's wife, Mary, recalls similarly how her knowledge of health and
health care allowed her to 'face up' to the certainty of his death:

I knew he wasn't going to make it -- let's face it he was really dead. It
was only his heart that was strong because he had a good heart for his
age and good lungs . . . I knew the first night they told me, and the
more I looked at him the more I knew . . . They did the best they could

for him, [everything] humanly possible, but his brain just wouldn't
heal up. His age was against him for a start, he was 74 though he
didn't look it

(From follow-up interview)

It is within this context of understanding, sense of involvement and prediction of death that the management and care of Mr Hart's body is interpreted. Mrs Hart, for example, recalled the importance to her of the nursing
care given to her husband, and how this not only protected her sense of
what was 'right' for Mr Hart as an individual, but how such care was
inextricably linked to her own sense of need and comfort. The following
extract concerns the period in which medical care had started to be withdrawn and death was openly acknowledged:

> *Mrs Hart*: they really cared for him and washed him and turned him,
> and another thing, they kept him shaved. I thought that was abso-
> lutely excellent.
> *JS*: Was that important to you?
> *Mrs Hart*: To me it was, and I think it was important to him as well.
> My husband was unconscious and unconscious people can't shave
> themselves. I can imagine that -- with shaving, you feel uncomfort-
> able and you feel dirty, and you know, Jack always shaved every
> day, he never missed a shave. I thought the standard of nursing was
> absolutely excellent . . . the care they gave him even when they knew.
> The nurses knew the same as I did that Jack wasn't going to come
> out of that coma, but they still treated him like a patient that was
> going to be alright, and washed him and shaved him . . . Looking
> after him . . . and lovely to me, so caring for me as well. [They] gave
> me a lot of support, the girls, without ever saying a great deal . . . In
> that intensive care, you felt as if they really care for you, you feel as
> though those nurses are really and truly caring for you the person
> and [that] they are putting their whole being, their whole self into
> caring for your man -- it were a very, very personal feeling and it
> made me feel comfortable.

(From follow-up interview)

The withdrawal of medical treatment from Mr Hart is construed similarly
to be supportive of his interests and in keeping with his own wishes. It is
seen also as in some way preserving his 'person', as a 'well', fit man, for
eternity:

> the only thing they could do was to discontinue treatment and just
> leave him alone [to] let him die in his own time . . . he's not going
> to suffer when he gets older with aches and pains, or go infirm and
> senile.

(From follow-up interview)

Such an interpretation sustains Michael and Mrs Hart across the course of Mr Hart's dying, in spite of his rather hurried transfer to a ward because of problems of bed availability and in spite of the marked changes in his appearance that develop as a result of the withdrawal of intravenous and naso-gastric fluids. In her final recollections of the moment of death, Mrs Hart's predominant memory is of peacefulness and of care:

> when he died we were there for a quarter of an hour after he took his last breath and he looked – to say a dead person looked nice – Jack really looked at peace. Yes, he didn't have a drawn face or a twisted down face. His face was just right. It was lovely, he really looked lovely. Those girls on [the] ward cared for him as well -- they were good nurses, very good nurses.
>
> (From follow-up interview)

I have drawn here a comparison between the deaths of two individuals and explored how the issues of predictability, understanding, and knowledge played a central role in the interpretation of the bodily care and management of these people. Several references have been made in the preceding discussion to the importance of trust in the relations between companions and healthcare staff. It has been suggested implicitly, by means of the re-peated reference to 'caring' behaviours, that the emergence of such trust depends on the development of a degree of emotional intimacy between these two parties. Where trust existed, then bodily care and management is interpreted as that which allows the *integration* of 'person' within body, in spite of the appearance of that body. Where trust was undermined, then bodily management and care is interpreted as encouraging the *disintegration* of 'person' within body. In the example of Mrs Stafford trust was undermined, in my interpretation, not only because of her family's lack of understanding about the seriousness of her condition, but also because of her movement from one surgical ward, to the intensive care unit and back to another surgical ward all in a relatively short period of time. Such dis-continuous, dislocated care meant that those relationships that were formed between healthcare staff and companions were of a fragile, episodic and non-sustainable nature.

In the next section we turn to further examine the importance of develop-ing 'close' relationships between healthcare staff and companions, relating attention to emotional 'need' of companions with the emergence within them of a sense of the trustworthiness of the healthcare staff.

Integrity of trust

During the follow-up interview with Michael Hart, he described his feelings regarding his relationship with the intensive care staff who had looked after his father as a 'kinship thing'. He recalled how he regretted the transfer of his father to the general ward for Michael's sake, rather than for any serious concerns about the quality of his father's care:

> You knew there were no more intensive care to be done with, no more medical help; but it's yourself you think about isn't it? You don't want to lose that [care], you don't want to leave -- It's hard to say what you felt, but you felt a bonding, a closeness that you didn't want to leave
>
> (From follow-up interview)

Michael recalled how this sense of intimacy developed as a result of the 'constant attention' that he received from the intensive care staff. He compared such attention to the feeling of desolation he had experienced on other occasions, in other areas of the hospital, which he likens to being 'at a bus stop with no bus coming'. Similarly, his mother recalled her sense of 'personal' attention and relates this to her belief that the intensive care staff were: 'really and truly caring for you the person . . . it made me feel as though they cared about what was happening' (follow-up interview).

This theme of 'kinship' and personal investment was visible in other cases, and was linked not only to the high level of visible 'care' giving, but also to a particular style of communication in which knowledge about medical technology and prognosis were 'shared', and personal feelings exchanged. The intensive care staff in both units often had to work hard to develop trust between themselves and patients' companions, especially in those circumstances where there was marked prognostic uncertainty and where the use of technology had to be explained repeatedly. These issues are explored below.

Expressions of trust and distrust

Mr Martin was a 74-year-old man admitted to intensive care in Western hospital for management of cardiogenic shock and pneumonia following emergency abdominal surgery. Shortly after admission to intensive care, surgery had to be repeated for bleeding, and so Mr Martin underwent two major operations within a few hours of each other. He spent 18 days in intensive care, before recovering sufficiently to be discharged to a ward. He eventually returned home after seven weeks in hospital and having been close to death on a number of occasions. A follow-up interview was carried out four months later involving his daughter Barbara and her husband Tom; and his son Philip and Philip's wife Carol. During the interview they described the course and severity of his illness and the prolonged period of uncertainty that they endured before his eventual recovery.

Throughout the account of Mr Martin's illness given by his family it is possible to trace a recurrent distrust of the explanations given by medical and nursing staff. This seems to stem from three sources:

1 an underlying cynicism they have about the motives of health professionals, which has derived from other experiences with the health service;
2 the length of time which they have to wait for explanations to be provided;
3 the way in which they perceived the explanations given as contradictory.

However, on occasions distrust gives way to an almost implicit faith. This seems to occur when they perceive that particular individuals have engaged with their concerns and anxieties and responded to them in a manner that indicates emotional reciprocity and an equitable exchange of knowledge. Again, as in the case of Mrs Stafford, overarching the whole account is a portrayal of the rapid 'processing' of an elderly person moved from place to place within the hospital. It is this 'processing' that seems to be at the root of the mistrust permeating the family's account. They have constantly to negotiate access to knowledge about his condition with various members of the healthcare staff with whom, in most cases, they have only fleeting contact. This episodic contact creates problems of assessment for the family since they are unable to judge the accuracy of the information with which they are provided. It is only when information is given by those with whom they feel some 'personal' connection that they develop any sense of 'trust' in that person and therefore in the validity of the information being provided. These themes are particularly vivid in Barbara's account of the difficulties she had in obtaining what she saw as 'reliable' information following her father's second operation, and during his first two days in intensive care:

> The next day, we stayed all night at the hospital again . . . personally I didn't think he would come round. Every time I went I was expecting the worst. He'd been in two or three days and we still wanted to know what this second operation was for, what was the cause of it – so we were there [waiting] for hours and hours. 'The doctor will see you at 11 o'clock' and no doctor arrives. Oh, hours and hours went past and we'd had no sleep, and eventually we insisted that we got to see the main man, I think it was Mr X, and he came in and said: 'What do you want to know, what do you know?' So we said that for a start the nurses on the other ward had said he had got an ulcer. He said: 'It's nothing whatever to do with that, on the general wards they do not always know everything. Sometimes they just class it as an ulcer.' So I said: 'Well, what's the cause of it?' and he said: 'It's just bad luck, just one of them things.' Anyhow, and I says: 'Will it come back again? Is it likely to happen again?' and he says: 'No, not necessarily,

you know, no reason why it should.' That was a relief . . . he said it were just bad luck.

(From follow-up interview)

We have a presentation here of a relatively matter of fact and unemotional response by the consultant surgeon to the family, whose members are in the grip of extreme anxiety and concern; the condition to which their father has almost succumbed on two occasions is presented as: 'just bad luck' and 'one of those things'. They ask for reassurance about reoccurrence and get a limited 'no reason why it should', which they accept as a source of relief and comfort. Barbara's brother, Philip, however remembered being 'put in [his] place' by the consultant surgeon and expressed his anger during the interview that his 'right' to knowledge about his father was not respected. This extract gives the impression of a struggle for ownership of knowledge about Mr Martin between the surgeon and Philip:

> I mean I like to ask people questions; oh, perhaps I shouldn't be asking these questions. This chap, Mr X, [the surgeon] I was asking questions and he sort of put me in my place. I was taken aback by it and I probably deserved it, but I wanted to know what was going on and I wanted the truth. He were really, he looked at me all snotty like and I thought *I have as much right to find out about my dad as anyone else!*

(From follow-up interview)

There is a marked contrast between the family's portrayal of the level of distrust with which they regarded the personnel from the 'ordinary' world of the hospital and the high levels of trust with which they regarded the intensive care staff. This trust, which was expressed as an almost fundamental faith, was mainly focused on one individual, but extended out to other members of the intensive care team. For example, Barbara's contrasting account of the events in intensive care demonstrates the level of trust that she and the rest of the family placed in one particular nurse, Mr Martin's named nurse 'Roy':

> *Barbara*: As I say, while he was up there and the nurses would explain this had happened and that has happened. One of the nurses, Roy, he were marvellous and he explained everything, anything we wanted to know. He really says to us, if time did come, you know, they'd tell us before they took his drips and that down, there is a hope you know.
>
> *JS*: What did that mean to you?
>
> *Barbara*: It meant hope, he give me hope . . . In that intensive care that nurse, Roy, everything he told us were true, you know like he told us about what was going to happen and everything he seemed to tell us, it seemed to happen. When one thing he told us came true, you

thought everything he said, and everything he did say, were true . . . I think the best thing about Roy was that he didn't just tell you the good things he'd tell you the bad things as well, and put you in the picture. You knew he was honest with you . . . Perhaps some people don't want to hear it, what could happen; perhaps it's just me, a person who likes to know.

(From follow-up interview)

The *way* in which Roy gave the information to Barbara and the rest of the family seemed to engender a sense of integrity and trustworthiness not present to the same extent in the other fleeting encounters that they had with various members of the healthcare staff. They remember the nurse becoming 'really emotional' at times and 'almost crying' such that he found it difficult to speak with them and relay news of their father's poor progress. Such expression of emotion made them feel that this nurse 'cared' for their father in a very personal way.

Other incidents in intensive care reinforced the family's belief in the trust-worthiness and competency of the staff there. Philip gives a particularly vivid example in his account of sitting beside his father and asking one of the anaesthetists to explain an X-ray to him. The willingness of the anaes-thetist to explain the X-ray to him, in spite of initial reluctance or surprise at the request, meant, for Philip, that he could 'keep in touch' and have a more tangible idea of his father's progress.[3] Philip gives a sense of feeling that he was being treated on an equal footing *vis à vis* the anaesthetist:

I was just sitting there and I've always been one for looking at the bottom of the charts and everything. I saw some, er, I saw some X-ray charts up on a screen and I asked the anaesthetist to explain it. And he looked at me gone out, as if to say, this is my job, this is nothing to do with you. He starts saying all about, you don't really understand what an X-ray is; I still don't I don't suppose, but it was like all fog and he says that was all fluid on his lungs, and I was asking him and he started to tell me, and keeping me in touch. But if I hadn't asked -- if you can actually see progress on an X-ray that he's getting a bit better, he was saying that there's no way he's out of the woods yet, he's still a long, long, way to go, but I [was able to see]

(From follow-up interview)

The focus in this example has demonstrated the importance of trust rela-tionships between healthcare staff and patients' companions during the acute uncertainty of critical illness and when death is highly likely to occur. It has shown that intensive care presented the opportunity for sustained contact between Mr Martin's family and a member of the healthcare staff, so that this continuous contact allowed them to develop a relationship of trust, which was reinforced by the intimate, 'personal' style in which they were given information regarding Mr Martin's condition. During this time they perceived also that their own fears and anxieties were being taken into account, as well as the emotional needs and insecurities of Mr Martin. It was this *integration* of emotional sensitivity with the apparently honest disclosure of information that engendered the conditions in which trust could develop. This was in marked contrast to the earlier episodic contacts that they had experienced and in which they judged that information had been both unreliable and delivered in an insensitive or uncaring manner.

Summary and discussion

The data examined here suggest that it is perceptions of the *meaning of* technology that determine representations of 'good' death in the intensive care unit. These perceptions, in their turn, depend crucially on the particular circumstances with which dying is attended, the purposes to which technology is employed by clinical staff, and the extent to which patients' companions are able to develop understanding and trust in these actions. Furthermore, the manner in which similar practices of bodily management can be construed as either supportive *or* unsupportive of 'personhood' captures how the representation of the 'good' death depends not only on the activities and intentions of the healthcare staff, but also on the motives attributed *to* them by the patients' companions who are the hyper-watchful observers of those activities. Linked inextricably to, and dependent on, these interpretations of motive is the emergence of conditions that facilitate open and honest communications between healthcare staff and patient's companions.

As Timmermans has noted (1998: 162) 'naive romanticized notions' of dying in pre-technological societies still hold considerable thrall over the representation of death in social science and healthcare literature and have led to an underexamination of the ways in which people in Western cultures incorporate now commonplace technology into their accounts of death. In particular, the sheer diversity of experience associated with death and the variety of sense and meaning created from these experiences tends to be neglected within the 'grand scheme' (Small 1997: 218) of demedicalization and anti-technology that underpins much contemporary death-related literature. The data presented here support a body of recent research (Kellehear 1990; Williams 1990; Seale 1995a,b; Bradbury 1996; Firth 1996; Payne *et al.* 1996; Young and Cullen 1996) which suggests that distinctive beliefs and ideas concerning the characteristics of the 'good' death elicited from lay respondents do not necessarily correspond to the predominant discourse of demedicalization espoused in death-related literature. Rather, the accounts of lay respondents show a warp and weft effect of ideas drawn from a variety of sources, combined such that medical intervention during dying is portrayed as sometimes supportive of an appropriate way to die and at other times in direct opposition to this. For example, Williams (1990), in a study of attitudes to death and illness among older people living in Aberdeen, found that his respondents possessed concepts of 'good' death that were drawn from a variety of cultural and historical influences. In a phrase that captures the range and complexity of ideas expressed about death and the 'right way to die', Williams describes how his respondents' attitudes to dying appear as: 'historical strata laid down by a culture in motion' (1990: 121). In these 'strata' potentially paradoxical ideas about the roles of nature, medicine, religion and self-determination are elided in contextually contingent ways that serve to represent particular values or experiences.

Calnan and Williams (1992, 1994) in the context of a broader study of public attitudes to modern medicine, note similarly the complexity and ambivalence of lay thinking in which views do not necessarily fall into the neat, logically consistent patterns suggested by popular models of discourse. Following Turner (1984), they suggest that the 'discourse determinism' implied by Foucault's theorization that medical discourse fashions the way in which we all think, perceive and speak about the body fails to provide space for the consideration of the phenomenology of embodiment and subjective experience. The data presented here suggest that it is within the phenomenology of suffering associated with the critical illness or death of a close companion that some insights may be gleaned of the relationship between individual experience and the representation of 'good' death and dying. The accounts presented here suggest that the memories with which death and near death are associated are subject to a process of interpretative construction and reconstruction, which continues long after the actual experience of the events themselves. Such a process has been characterized as a 'resurrective practice' (Seale 1995b: 378) in which the speaker reduces the threat of death to a personal 'ontological security' (Giddens 1991: 3) by a narrative and reflexive reworking of events.

In this chapter, we have seen how the practices associated with modern medicine have become an 'abstract system' or 'creed', which we *trust* to perform according to deeply ingrained and almost unconscious expectations (Giddens 1990, 1991; Lupton 1994; Williams and Calnan 1996). This would appear to be a pivotal element of the 'good' death in the highly technological confines of the modern intensive care unit. The maintenance of this trust is, however, conjoined with the risk of disillusion and crushing disappointment on those occasions when these deeply held beliefs are thwarted during the course of interactions with the medical world: 'lay views towards science and technology, including modern medicine, come to comprise a shifting dialectic of trust and doubt, certainty and uncertainty, reverence and disillusionment. Medicine, in short, becomes a fountain of hope and font of despair as its 'limitations' are exposed as never before' (Williams and Calnan 1996: 1613).

Notes

1 Data regarding family members' prospective expectations and understandings regarding patients' prognosis were recorded in observational field notes following informal conversations with the author.
2 Clearly, a potential fourth pattern exists: expectation of life/life as the outcome. However, none of the participants' experiences fell into this category, and this is therefore not discussed.
3 Interestingly the family misinterprets the role of the anaesthetic staff, seeing them not as doctors but as clever technicians or theatre staff. The misinterpretation is revealed where Tom and Philip are explaining to me the extent of their father's illness:

Tom: Everything went, his lungs, his kidneys packed up, his liver packed up, and he had a heart attack didn't he?
Philip: That's what they do up there isn't it? I didn't realize how clever those anaesthetists are!
Tom: Oh, they were (really) nice blokes those anaesthetists, never too much trouble for them to explain.
Philip: We didn't see doctors, it were all those in green that were looking after him. They were more caring the staff in there, the anaesthetists, than the flipping doctors.

(From retrospective interview)

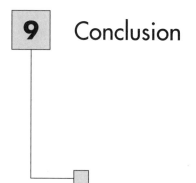

9 Conclusion

Social action surrounding critically ill people in intensive care is, in many ways, on 'fast forward'. In a time span covering only a few days or weeks, people are admitted, diagnosed, investigated, discussed and cared for until their death or recovery. During this time, inter-professional activity can be frenetic and fast moving. Clinical knowledge must be produced about the ill person; relationships formed and sustained among healthcare staff, patients and patients' companions. Further, the technological environment of intensive care and its relationship to the highly segmented hospital organization allows some conclusions to be drawn about the impact of the 'hyper-specialization' of contemporary health care on the management of ill and dying people. I have sought to slow down and dwell on the complexity of social action in intensive care. Moreover, I have tried to reveal this as *it occurs*, rather than merely relying on individuals' retrospective accounts of these processes. In so doing we have been able to explore the trajectory of critical illness from shortly after admission to intensive care to beyond death or recovery.

A central theme throughout the book has been the treatment of decision making as a social process bounded by particular organizational contexts, rather than a product of individual reasoning governed by immutable ethical and scientific principles. Such principles *are* present, but are revealed here as being subject to interpretation and re-interpretation during social interaction. Within this social analysis of decision making in intensive care, attention has focused specifically on the management of the ill person's body. The critically ill people in this study were unconscious and as such had, at first sight, no control or agency over events determining their care. However, their body was *constitutive of* other's 'work', with the nature of 'body' and of such work being the subjects of potential dispute and conflict.

The presence of the 'material body' in this data, and the evidence of its profound influence on the character of social interaction, addresses a space within sociological theory (Turner 1996). Here we are able to see how the 'body' as a corporeal reality impinges on the socially constructive work of medicine. Rather than the 'body without organs' (Fox 1993: 24), which is discursively malleable in almost infinite ways, the 'body with organs' is shown to play an active role in constraining and directing the clinical discourse of which it is a subject. Further, in this analysis, medicine is revealed as enacted by thinking, feeling individuals who may, at times, actively resist the conforming pressures of mainstream clinical ideology.

Chapter 3 picked up this particular theme with an analysis of how diagnostic and prognostic certainty was achieved about the health history and quality of life of individuals admitted to intensive care. In a discussion that focused on the compilation of negotiated accounts of the body, the way in which clinical data is assembled, read, and interpreted during group activities was examined. A particular emphasis was placed in this chapter on the difficult tasks of unravelling the complex problems of elderly, chronically ill individuals in the face of a number of possible interpretations concerning their previous and potential state of health. The role of the ward round and the use of the medical notes as routines that enable the delimitation and structuring of medical action were highlighted in this discussion. The use of these routines gives some insight in turn into the complex processes of 'micro-rationing' (Hughes and Griffiths 1997), which occur within intensive care and without which difficult clinical choices could not be made.

Chapter 4 focused more closely on nursing and medical work in intensive care. A particular emphasis in this chapter was the delineation of contradictory elements in nursing work in intensive care which, it was argued, become especially problematic to manage as critically ill individuals move towards death. Nursing work was presented as being constituted dually, first by the medical-technical approach of medicine and second by strategies directed towards the incorporation of the 'whole person' into a focus that threatens to be essentially depersonalized. This chapter also showed how nurses' attention to the medical-technical aspects of their role ensures that they express conflict with medical staff concerning the management of dying patients in an oblique fashion. Essentially, nurses recognize the constraints faced by medical staff in basing action on any footing other than 'technological'. Further, they recognize that the technological recognition of dying *lags behind* the acknowledgement of that state as a material fact.

Chapter 5 looked at the extent to which patients' companions are involved in the process of planning care decisions. The emphasis here was on methods by which staff give information to companions; on the various ways in which companions *use and interpret* that information; and on their recollections of this aspect of their experience. Some indication was given in this discussion of potential barriers to the formation of trusting and reciprocal relationships between staff and companions.

Chapter 6 further developed the theme of mismatched dying trajectories introduced in Chapter 4, with an analysis of the withdrawal of active medical treatment from dying patients. Here the focus was on *how* a withdrawal of medical treatment is effected in intensive care. The discussion demonstrated how medical work is constituted by strategies to ensure that clinical action is based on *technical* data rather than on *intuitive* clinical judgements. An examination was presented of how responsibility for treatment decisions is diffused and how problems of definition between euthanasia, withdrawal, and 'natural' death are overcome. This chapter argued that the difficulties that clinicians face during the course of their everyday work with critically ill and dying people must be allowed to further inform our thinking about the 'modern myth' of natural death (Hopkins 1997).

Chapter 7 was an exploration of how 'nursing care only' is constituted during and after the withdrawal of active medical treatment. Here it was suggested that nurses align 'body work' with 'emotional work' in order to reproduce the 'personhood' or individuality of their unconscious, dying patients. In this way, in spite of the technological environment of intensive care, the process of dying can often be invested with an atmosphere of almost familial intimacy and meaning. This analysis contributes to the whole debate about the nature of nursing work in which processes leading to 'knowing' the patient and the incorporation of the 'subjective' have been highlighted.

Chapter 8 moved on to examine the narrative reconstruction of events in intensive care by the companions of the patients, around whom the entire study focused. It explored the concept of the 'good death' and its applicability to deaths that occur in, or shortly after, intensive care. The concept of good death was reformulated in this chapter as a form of 'integrity' within which three interrelated dimensions were identified. These were presented as first, the maintenance of the 'natural order' by a resolution of the tension between 'nature' and 'technology' within intensive care; second, the maintenance of the 'personhood' of the dying individual; and third, the attention to the needs of companions for emotional support and trust. This chapter showed how human endeavours such as medical technology, determine 'natural death' in that they frame our very expectations and beliefs about *the way things should be, or should have been.* In the discussion of personhood, the *meaning* for the companions of bodily care of the ill patients was emphasized, showing how particular styles of bodily care and management are critical in the preservation of the 'person' of ill individuals who may appear, in their unconscious state, to be *already dead.* In such situations, it was argued, the representation of 'person' depends not only on the activities and agency of the healthcare staff but also on the motives attributed to them by the ill patient's companions who are the hyper-watchful observers of those actions.

Returning to the earlier theme of the relationships between staff and companions raised in Chapter 5, Chapter 8 shows that the existence of trust is pivotal to the interpretation of bodily management as supportive of personhood. Key features, which encourage the development of trusting relationships, were identified as responses to the emotional needs of companions, the sharing and exchange of information and knowledge and the expression of personal feelings. Trust was shown to be fundamentally undermined in those instances where companions experienced the care delivered to the patient as fragmented or in some way inconsistent with their understanding of the nature of the patient's illness. This may have occurred during events leading up to an individual's admission to intensive care, or during the period of post-intensive care management. In some cases, companions were able to describe fleeting or episodic contact with numerous members of healthcare staff in various areas of the hospital. The temporary and unsustained nature of such contacts meant that companions found themselves in the position of having to renegotiate access to knowledge about the patient as well as having to make difficult judgements about the validity of information that was sometimes perceived as contradictory. The importance of intensive care staff giving appropriate explanantions about the use of technology and in a manner that neither assumes prior understanding nor patronizes the intelligence of patients' companions, is clearly highlighted in Chapter 8. This echoes other recent commentaries on this subject (Stroud 1997; Fulbrook *et al.* 1999a,b,c).

Implications for nursing and healthcare practice

In many ways the healthcare staff within intensive care carry an awesome responsibility to match, or counter, the pervasive images of 'intensive care' that are represented in the media and absorbed by the rest of us. These are images which include not only the 'best' of medical care, that which is relied on in the crisis and fear of acute illness when rapid, competent action is needed to restore health and life; but also the 'worst' of medical care, the medical or technical mistake, the exclusion of humanity and individual control or the prolongation of death by means of impersonal machinery. Further, intensive care is at the apex of a system of hospital organization that is increasingly specialized and isolated. Such a system, it may be argued, is poorly suited to providing a comprehensive, co-ordinated or multi-disciplinary response to the complicated end-of-life needs of an increasingly elderly, socially disadvantaged, and chronically ill population (Gordon and Singer 1995; Dunnell 1997; Debate of the Age Health and Care Study Group 1999).

That intensive care suffers the consequences for an overall reluctance to embrace these issues is highlighted in this book. The case studies have shown all too clearly how people can, as if by accident, end up in intensive care having aggressive and inappropriate treatment. This is not because of negligence, incompetence or inhumanity. In fact the opposite is true. Individual staff are shown in this study as facing almost intolerably difficult judgements to act in the patient's best interest. These are judgements that have to be made quickly and often with recourse to little or no previous knowledge regarding that person. This is a problem alluded to by authors such as Jennett (1984, 1994), in analyses of the problems currently endemic in the treatment of critical illness in elderly people. At the time of the field work both intensive care units had guidelines (albeit at differing levels of specificity) to aid staff in the identification of those patients who can best be helped by intensive care. However, partly due to the issues of knowledge and information alluded to already, these were of limited use. Since the completion of the field work, guidelines on admission have been developed at a national level (Department of Health 1996), in response to a nation-wide survey that found that one in six referrals to intensive care is inappro-priate (Metcalfe and McPherson 1994). The impact of these guidelines has yet to be assessed, but it may be that such 'top-down' approaches do little to alleviate problems rooted deep within the structure and culture of West-ern health care.

The situation in which intensive care becomes responsible for the dis-entanglement of end-of-life problems causes acute difficulties for medical and nursing staff as they attempt to care for dying people in a humane and appropriate way. It also engenders potential confusion in their relation-ships with the ill patient's companions. Companions have varying responses depending on their perception of the situation. For example, they may believe that 'intensive care' is a particular sort of modern day saviour, only to feel let down, angry and grief stricken when their husband, wife, partner or child eventually dies, especially if intensive care has been withdrawn and the death of that person occurs elsewhere in the hospital. They may feel disempowered because of a sudden, inexplicable, input of 'technology' when they believed that an expected death was imminent. Of course, such experi-ences of loss and bereavement are not exclusive to those who have con-tact with intensive care, they are a feature of 'normal' patterns of grieving following deaths in other situations. However, they are a central and recurring feature of life in intensive care: problems that have to be faced and resolved on an almost daily basis.

The way in which healthcare delivery is currently structured is, it may be argued, at the root of such problems. The 'acute care culture', depicted here, depends on a hospital organization structured around finding solu-tions to *immediate*, short-term health problems. This is done primarily by means of gathering a series of 'specialist' opinions, each of which focuses on a particular aspect of 'the patient'. Decisions are then made on the basis of information that becomes progressively narrower and less contextual in nature, and the threat of death is contained, postponed and deconstructed into a series of potentially soluble puzzles (Illich 1976; Bauman 1992, Moller 1996). What occurs is a cascade of decisions (Slomka 1992), in which there are a myriad of contributors, each of whom believes that their version of 'the patient' is the most cogent. The clinical ownership of patients by particular 'firms' directs the gathering of specialist opinions; the value of which are adjudicated according to judgements that are presented as purely technical. Accordingly, the wider social and human issues are often either ignored, alluded to only in passing, or seen as introducing murky irrationality into the whole medical enterprise. At the time of the field work, the pressure imposed on clinicians to operate within a market system of health care (Department of Health 1989) encouraged such tightly focused activity and was clearly acting as a disincentive to taking a more discursive, *social* approach to the management of patients. As Paris and Reardon have stated: 'most critically and terminally ill patients continue to be cared for in institutions in which aggressive intervention and the treatment of acute episodes is the norm' (1991: 1933). In the extract below, Moller refers to what he later describes as the 'roller coaster journey' of the patient who is eventually designated as dying:

> the technical care of dying patients enables physicians and other medical staff to treat the dying patient with the same set of expectations and responses applied to other medical patients. It is for this reason that dying patients with a lingering trajectory are often cast in the sick role, and attention is focused primarily on the management of physical symptoms. By focusing on the manageability of symptoms, the unmanageability of dying is superseded and deferred. As a result the process of dying is prolonged in such a way that it is often filled with uncertainty and ambivalence
>
> (Moller 1996: 68)

Another aspect to this problem is a lack of knowledge among surgeons and physicians about how to care effectively for older people with complex illnesses. A recent inquiry reveals that many patients receive suboptimal care before admission to intensive care (McQuillan *et al*. 1998). Suboptimal care has been linked in turn to the observation that the greatest percentage of deaths in the UK intensive care unit is in patients admitted from the hospital wards (Goldhill and Sumner 1998). As Goldhill *et al*. note in a letter to the *British Medical Journal* patients admitted from the wards to the intensive care unit 'are likely to represent the tip of the iceberg of preventable deaths on the ward . . . others with potentially treatable conditions may be deteriorating on the wards beyond the point where admission to intensive care can be of benefit' (1998: 195).

Intensive care units, then, grapple increasingly with the legacy of the failure of that wider system to come to terms with the changing face of illness and death in modern societies. It is beyond the remit of this conclusion to attempt to address comprehensively the vast range of concerns that come into play here. It is clear that they will not be solved by any simple combination of interventions. Moreover the scale of the problem appears such that *any* recommendations will fail to influence the basic context and environment within which intensive care is placed. Notwithstanding these qualifications, there may be new approaches and practices that can be incorporated into current clinical routines and education by means of relatively small adaptations. These would go some way to addressing some of the problems that beset the care of critically ill and dying people within intensive care as well as in the wider hospital environment. Three groups of suggestions are focused on below: (1) the creation of some continuity between intensive care and the wider healthcare system; (2) the enhancement of teamwork and staff support within intensive care; and (3) the re-examination of the involvement, participation and support of companions and families during the process of care decision making, as well as in the period following death and critical illness.

Enabling continuity of care

At many points in the foregoing discussion the issue of 'continuity' of care across the healthcare system is revealed as problematic. This has significant effects on both the development of treatment plans for individual patients first admitted into intensive care from other areas of the hospital and on the perceptions of their companions regarding the purpose, direction and quality of care. One aspect to this, examined in Chapter 3, is the limited, immediate availability of comprehensive information regarding the patient's health history and quality of life. This constrains the ability of clinicians to develop treatment plans and, in the cases examined, leads to an apparent over-use of intensive therapies in patients who are reaching the end of a course of chronic illness. The attempt to compile a profile of the health history and quality of life of each patient is shown as an ongoing feature of clinical work in intensive care, but one that features particularly strongly in the preliminary assessment of patients. This study suggests that such information is crucial in determining not only the extent of treatment given to an individual but, more fundamentally, the initial placement of patients in intensive care. Several of the case studies illustrate a scenario in which the extent of an individual's chronic illness and disability is not discovered until very substantial intensive therapies have been commenced. Further, the perceptions of their companions regarding the appropriateness of those interventions are not explored comprehensively until after such treatments have been initiated. As shown in Chapter 6, once such therapies are commenced, it is only by dint of complicated interactional work that they can be withdrawn: this is in spite of the contemporary ethical position that maintains no essential difference between the withholding of 'futile' treatments and the 'withdrawal' of such treatments once instigated (Randall and Downie 1996; BMA 1999).

The other aspect to the problem of continuity concerns the organization of medical and nursing work across the hospital site; and the way in which care is planned and co-ordinated predominantly *within* individual wards and intensive care units, rather than *across* those organizational boundaries. This issue is examined in Chapter 8, in an analysis of the perceptions of companions regarding the nursing care and medical treatment of patients during the whole course of that individual's critical illness. Recurrent themes identified here concern the perception of the movement from intensive care to the general wards as transfer from 'rich to poor' in terms of the contrast between the level and quality of nursing and medical care and an interpretation of that care as confusing and inconsistent in terms of its overall purpose.

This transfer of patients from intensive care to a general ward highlights a particular problem. In some cases patients were clearly going to die in the short term, while in other cases patients had been designated as not likely to benefit from further intensive therapy, i.e. as likely to die in the medium or long term. When this occurred it was often because of limited bed availability, but it led to an exacerbation of confusion and regret over the delivery of care expressed by patient's companions. While companions understood the need for transfer, they expressed regret at losing the attentive nursing care that intensive care could provide to the dying person, and the emotional support they had gained from the formation of close relationships with the nurses primarily responsible for the patient.

Models of practice are available, which could be adapted to address these problems. In the SUPPORT study, for example, an intervention was designed by researchers to improve the level of information available to physicians about the prognoses of patients. The intervention had three components. First, a brief written report regarding a patient's probability of surviving for a six-month period, likelihood of being severely functionally impaired at two months, and probability of surviving cardiopulmonary resuscitation. Second, a written report was provided regarding the patient's views on cardiopulmonary resuscitation, treatment preferences, and perceived prognosis. These reports were prepared by the researchers. Third, specially trained nurse facilitators were given responsibility for initiating and maintaining communication among patients, their companions and the healthcare staff.

Such initiatives could be helpful in informing decision making particularly in the case of those patients whose referral for admission to intensive care follows a period of treatment elsewhere in the hospital organization. It may also be possible to incorporate some aspects of the first two stages of the intervention into the information recorded about elderly and chronically ill patients in the primary care setting, although this presumes that such patients have had regular, close contact with their general practice prior to the onset of an acute exacerbation of their condition. That this is not necessarily the case is an indicator of the extent of the information gap that needs to be addressed. Enhancing the quality and range of information from primary care would, however, be a necessary component in informing the very rapid process of decision making that takes place around critically ill patients admitted from home to hospital via a general practitioner referral.

The SUPPORT study (Principal Investigators for the SUPPORT Project 1995) showed, however, that the mere provision of information did not alter the treatment preferences of physicians and that the role of nurses during the third part of the intervention was problematic. Lo (1995) suggests that the intervention did not address the wider organizational and cultural issues in which the autonomy and accountability of *individual* physicians remains central to the process of care decision making. This encourages physicians to rely on judgements informed by their own expertise rather than on judgements made by others (such as nurses), since they may be perceived as less accountable for patient care. Further, this encourages a narrow, biomedical interpretation of prognosis and 'quality of life', which may not correspond to perspectives held by nurses, families or primary care staff, and which disallows an incorporation of those perspectives into an evaluation of what constitutes an appropriate course of action.

The issue of responsibility for care would appear to be central here. Nolan (1995: 305) suggests that for any movement to be made from a multi-disciplinary to an interdisciplinary model (in which a variety of perspectives contribute equally to the direction of clinical care and decision making), a willingness to share responsibility must be shown. This must come not only from doctors but also from nurses, who traditionally have deferred to their medical colleagues, particularly in difficult end-of-life discussions. Henneman *et al.* (1995: 359) suggest that many barriers to interdisciplinary collaboration can be traced to the socialization and education of nurses in which, in a similar way to doctors, independence rather than interdependence has been emphasized.

Several initiatives have been developed that may be used to address the problems of interdisciplinary work *across* ward boundaries. These include, for example, the move towards the creation of clinical nurse specialists and 'nurse consultants', which, it is suggested, will enable expertise to be shared across organizational boundaries (Wright 1992; Coyne 1996; Hall-Smith *et al.* 1997). The 'case management' model (Petryshen and Petryshen 1992; Hale 1995; Tahan 1999) is another innovation that features the involvement of a 'case manager' who monitors and co-ordinates a patient's episode of illness with the primary nurse(s), doctors and other staff. Commentators suggest that continuity of nursing and medical care may be enhanced by such initiatives, with the planning of care focusing on patient and companion need rather than occurring as a haphazard reaction to the short-term flux of bed availability and other organizationally driven pressures (Scholes *et al.* 1999). Ritter *et al.* (1992) report on a case management model, which could be adapted for use in critical care areas and in which major constituents of the charge nurse/sister role become that of liaison across organizational and occupational boundaries, and long-term planning for patient placement post-intensive care.

One example will be given here of an innovation in care that focuses specifically on the management of patients designated as dying within intensive and acute care settings. Reporting on experience of a 10-year 'end of life' service in a University hospital in Detroit, US, Campbell and Frank (1997) describe the establishment of a nurse-led palliative care service, which has served the acute care providers. This service shares some features with hospital palliative care services in this country. However, rather than being predominantly advisory and concerned with patients suffering mainly from malignancy, Campbell and Frank assume responsibility for the direction and planning of the care of all patients referred to them. They exercise this responsibility by conducting shared 'rounds' and by liaising closely with other medical and nursing staff responsible for implementing care. Patient referrals come largely from the medical intensive care unit, from the accident and emergency department, or from the acute medical and surgical departments. Where patients are referred from intensive care, Campbell and Frank become involved in, and facilitate, withdrawal of treatment discussions held with patients' companions and with intensive care staff. Further, they assume responsibility for the transfer and placement of patients to suitable non-intensive care areas. Once transfer has been completed, an interdisciplinary 'therapeutic plan' is instituted for each patient, in which nursing and medical goals are coalesced. Campbell and Frank report that the service has been a viable 'triage' option for the medical intensive care unit in the management of dying patients: allowing intensive care beds to be vacated and significant cost savings, but at the same time, ensuring high quality nursing and medical care to those who are dying and their companions.

Enhancing teamwork and staff support within intensive care

There were marked differences between the two intensive care units studied in terms of their approach to interdisciplinary collaboration. At Eastern, substantial moves have been made towards the development of 'nursing led' care. This is effected by means of a refashioning of the traditionally consultant-led ward round and by means of the introduction of primary nursing. Primary nursing at Eastern had been in operation for more than a year at the start of this study, while the reorganization of the ward round occurred during the period of fieldwork. The ward round became, during this time, nurse led, with the patient's 'case' and progress being presented to the rest of the staff by his or her nurse. An evaluation of a similar innovation within an intensive care unit is available (Wright *et al.* 1996), showing that nurses became more actively involved in care planning as a result.

At Western, nursing care is more fragmented. Although the named nurse system was in operation, patients do not always receive care from 'their' nurse in a consistent fashion. Further, collaboration between nursing and medical staff appears, in my interpretation, to be a function of individual personality and knowledge rather than a feature fostered actively by organizational procedures. The ward round at Western sometimes occurs with only incidental consultation and involvement of the nurse caring for the patient. The case studies of Mrs Hall (Chapters 3, 4 and 7) and Mr Randall from Western (Chapters 3 and 7) demonstrate in a particularly clear way that there are thus fewer *formal* opportunities to resolve issues of interdisciplinary conflict at Western than at Eastern.

In spite of these differences, staff in both units emphasize the importance of the 'team' in the delivery of care to patients. The introduction of primary nursing and the nurse-led ward round at Eastern has gone some way to addressing the tension between 'hierarchy and collegiality' (Griffiths 1997: 60) and thus made 'team' a viable term for describing the organization of action. However, at Western, the term seems to be applied more as a 'loose rubric than a detailed template for action' (Griffiths 1997: 60). Chapter 3 pointed out, however, that the reliance on the medical model during the ward round at Eastern means that the nursing orientation to patients is frequently subsumed to a requirement to produce a proficient medical report. While this is undoubtedly appropriate for those patients for whom recovery is still expected, it is problematic for those patients who are approaching death even if this has not been acknowledged formally. Further, nurses' anxieties about their 'grasp' of medical data appears to constrain them from making their opinions known *vis à vis* treatment plans for patients. Another aspect to this was revealed in Chapter 7, when it was shown that once a patient has been designated formally as beyond the help of 'medicine', doctors are often only minimally involved with their care and nurses were sometimes left in a position of uncertainty regarding the management of an individual's death. The analysis of 'nursing' in this book shows the practical and emotional difficulties this can involve. The moving descriptions from nurses themselves and from the most intimate observers of nursing care, the families and companions of patients reveal how very well placed intensive care is to give attentive, loving care to those approaching death. Such care is remembered with gratitude by families and companions, playing a central role in their accounts of death. However, there is a high risk that the opposite may occur. Crucially, the success of nursing in this regard seems to depend on the emergence of a shared understanding with medicine.

Several adaptations could be made to current practices that may consolidate the progressive and effective changes introduced by Eastern intensive care unit. These may help to develop a more interdisciplinary perspective, which would be especially valuable in managing the care of dying patients and their companions. Shared shift patterns may be one approach to forging interdisciplinary links, since these would allow for shared, regularly repeated handovers of care. Another approach would be to complement the 'primary' nurse model by a similar approach to the allocation of medical care. Thus, rather than one of three or four consultants assuming responsibility for all the patients on a rotating pattern, each would assume responsibility for the care of perhaps only two of those individuals. They would thus forge closer links with each primary nurse and would co-ordinate the work of the more junior medical staff accordingly.

A further way of enhancing both interdisciplinary understanding, effectiveness and mutual support may be an adaptation of team debriefing after the death or discharge of patients. McNamara *et al.* (1994: 234) describe the operation of a 'separation review' in a palliative care context. This consists of a weekly, multi-disciplinary meeting in which the circumstances of the illness, care and death of a patient are discussed. Several questions guide the format of the review: whether those particular circumstances could be regarded as 'satisfactory' from the point of view of the patients, as well as their family/companions, and from the various positions of the healthcare teams. Such a model, if carefully adapted, may allow for cross-disciplinary evaluation of care, act as a form of clinical supervision *and* an opportunity for education. Similar models of 'debriefing' have been used in accident and emergency departments (Cudmore 1996), particularly for use after the resuscitation of patients. In such environments debriefing is seen as a *structured* opportunity to defuse stress after critical incidents and therefore offset the long-term risk of development of post-traumatic stress disorder and 'burnout' (Boyle *et al.* 1991; Farrington 1997).

Re-examining the involvement of companions during care decision making

Chapters 5 and 8 showed that communication between intensive care staff and patients' companions is predicated on a perceived need to 'warn' of the likelihood of death. Emphasis was placed on the role of the medical staff in delivering a formal presentation to companions regarding the condition of patients. In this formal presentation, efforts are made to stress the pessimistic aspects of an individual's prognosis. Nurses regard themselves as playing an important role in 'preparing' companions for this presentation and for the eventual death of a patient. Considerable energies are invested in facilitating the expression of grief and in developing a state akin to 'anticipatory grief' (Lindemann 1944) within companions. Furthermore, healthcare staff, who were interviewed, expressed the belief that families and companions should not be expected to assume responsibility for decisions regarding the continuation of care for patients. Rather, such an expectation was seen as placing an unfair burden on companions and as leading to a risk of 'abnormal' grieving in the future.

In some cases, however, this attention to the promotion of anticipatory grief, and to the removal of responsibility for care decisions from companions, may be misplaced. What has been seen, particularly in Chapter 5, is first, a variable tension between vulnerability and control within companions (Lupton 1996); and second, a very individual response to the prospect of death. Cray (1989) gives an example of how room for such individual variation might be addressed in a description of a family intervention programme in a medical intensive care unit. In this programme, special attention was given to the balancing of structured, routine approaches to the information needs of families and their individual circumstances. In this model, a clinical nurse specialist acted as a facilitator; in much the same way as reported by Campbell and Frank (1997) and Ritter *et al.* (1992) cited above. While this may be seen as an infringement of the role of the primary nurse, it would alleviate some of the problems reported by nurses in this study, where they described being 'torn' between the needs of their patient and the often very considerable demands and needs of that patient's companions for information and support. Further, it would ensure that specialist education could be targeted at the key individuals undertaking these roles. These individuals could then assume a counselling role directed at facilitating mutual understanding in a way that nurses at the bedside may not be able, or willing, to undertake. Such an individual could act as a supportive resource for companions and families both during the experience of critical illness and afterwards. Bereavement and critical illness follow-up could then be carried out with companions/families in a way that may not be practicable or desirable for patient-focused nurses (Jackson 1996). Such an intervention could be targeted to identify those most in need of follow up, following an approach identified by Kissane *et al.* (1996). This model creates an opportunity to move beyond a narrow definition of 'needs' encouraged both by the understandable tendency for staff under stress to follow 'routine' procedures and the continued reliance on research findings based on a 'tick-box' inventory of people's feelings.

These three suggestions are not intended as simple recipes for action. Rather they are 'food for thought' for those involved in the stressful and demanding processes of delivering care to critically ill and dying people. Further research will be required to elucidate and evaluate the most appropriate approaches to the care of such patients and their companions. This study has, it is hoped, made some contribution to that process. The primary motive behind this research has not been criticism, but rather the development of knowledge and understanding to help practitioners to alleviate the suffering that remains part and parcel of the modern healthcare environment. I hope that I have also added a small further force of leverage on the gradually opening sociological 'window' on death, dying and end-of-life decision making.

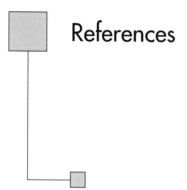

References

Ahronheim, J.C., Morrison, R.S., Baskin, S.A., Morris, J. and Meier, D.E. (1996) Treatment of the dying in the acute care hospital: advanced dementia and metastatic cancer. *Archives of Internal Medicine*, 156: 2094–100.

Airedale NHS Trust v *Bland*, 19 February 1993, 2 *Weekly Law Reports*: 316–400.

Ambiavagar, M. and McConn, R. (1978) Intensive therapy: a modern necessity. *Surgical Clinics of North America*, 58: 1031–44.

Anspach, R. (1987) Prognostic conflict in life and death decisions: the organization as an ecology of knowledge. *Journal of Health and Social Behaviour*, 28: 215–31.

Anspach, R. (1988) Notes on the sociology of medical discourse: the language of case presentation. *Journal of Health and Social Behaviour*, 29: 357–75.

Anspach, R. (1993) *Deciding Who Lives: Fateful Choices In the Intensive Care Nursery*. Berkley, CA: University of California Press.

Ariès, P. (1976) *Western Attitudes Towards Death: From the Middle Ages to the Present*. London: John Hopkins University Press.

Ariès, P. (1981) *The Hour of Our Death*. Allen Lane: London.

Armstrong, D. (1983a) *Political Anatomy of the Body: Medical Knowledge in Britain in the Twentieth Century*. Cambridge: Cambridge University Press.

Armstrong, D. (1983b) The fabrication of nurse-patient relationships. *Social Science and Medicine*, 17: 457–60.

Arney, W.R. and Bergen, B.J. (1984) *Medicine and the Management of Living*. Chicago, IL: University of Chicago Press.

Ashby, M. (1998) Palliative care, death causation, public policy and the law. *Progress in Palliative Care*, 6: 69–77.

Atkinson, P. (1981) *The Clinical Experience: The Construction and Reconstruction of Medical Reality*. Farnborough: Gower.

Atkinson, P. (1984) Training for certainty. *Social Science and Medicine*, 19: 949–56.

Atkinson, P. (1992) The ethnography of a medical setting: reading, writing and rhetoric. *Qualitative Health Research*, 2: 451–74.

Atkinson, P. (1995) *Medical Talk and Medical Work: The Liturgy of the Clinic.* London: Sage.

Atkinson, S., Bihari, D., Smithies, M. *et al.* (1994) Identification of futility in intensive care. *Lancet,* 344: 1203–6.

Audit Commission (1991) *The Virtue of Patients: Making Best Use of Ward Nursing Resources.* London: Audit Commission.

Audit Commission (1992) *Making Time for Patients: A Handbook for Ward Sisters.* London: Audit Commission.

Audit Commission (1999) *Critical to Success: The Place of Efficient and Effective Critical Care Services Within the Acute Hospital.* London: Audit Commission.

Baldock, G.J. (1995) Intensive care medicine in the reformed National Health Service (Editorial). *Anaesthesia,* 50: 671–3.

Baltz, J. and Wilson, J.L. (1995) Age-based limitation for ICU care: is it ethical? *Critical Care Nurse,* 15: 65–73.

Bauman, Z. (1992) *Mortality, Immortality and Other Life Strategies.* Oxford: Polity.

Bayliss, R. (1982) Thou shalt not strive officiously. *British Medical Journal,* 285: 1373–4.

Benner, P. and Wrubel, J. (1989) *The Primacy of Caring: Stress and Coping in Health and Illness.* Menlo Park, CA: Addison-Wesley.

Benner, P., Tanner, C.A. and Chesla, C.A. (1996) *Expertise in Nursing Practice: Caring, Clinical Judgement and Ethics.* New York: Springer.

Bennett, D. (1995) *Doctors Call for More Intensive Care Beds and Nurses* (Press Release). London: St George's NHS Trust.

Bennett, P. (1995) Cutting the thread of life: legal guidelines for the withdrawal of treatment following the Anthony Bland case. *Critical Care Medicine,* 11: 62–4.

Berg, M. (1992) The construction of medical disposals: medical sociology and medical problem solving in clinical practice. *Sociology of Health and Illness,* 14: 151–80.

Bion, J. (1995) Rationing intensive care. *British Medical Journal,* 310: 682–3.

Bion, J. and Strunin, L. (1996) Multiple organ failure: from basic science to prevention (Editorial). *British Journal of Anaesthesia,* 77: 1–2.

Blackburn, A.M. (1989) Problems of terminal care in elderly patients. *Palliative Medicine,* 3: 203–6.

Bloor, M. (1976) Bishop Berkley and the adeno-tonsillectomy enigma. *Sociology,* 10: 43–61.

Bloor, M. (1978a) On the analysis of observational data: a discussion of the worth and uses of inductive techniques and respondent validation. *Sociology,* 12: 545–57.

Bloor, M. (1978b) On the routinised nature of work in people-processing agencies: the case of adenotonsillectomy assessments in ENT out-patient clinics, in A. Davis (ed.) *Relationships between Doctors and Patients.* Farnborough: Gower.

Bloor, M. and McIntosh, J. (1990) Surveillance and concealment: a comparison of techniques of client resistance in therapeutic communities and health visiting, in S. Cunningham-Burley and N. McKeganey (eds) *Readings in Medical Sociology.* London: Routledge.

Bond, S. (1983) Nurses' communications with cancer patients, in J. Wilson-Barnett (ed.) *Nursing Research: Ten Studies in Patient Care.* Chichester: Wiley.

Bosk, C.L. (1979) *Forgive and Remember: Managing Medical Failure.* Chicago, IL: University of Chicago Press.

Bowden, P. (1997) *Caring: Gender Sensitive Ethics*. London: Routledge.

Bowers, L. (1989) The significance of primary nursing. *Journal of Advanced Nursing*, 14: 13–19.

Boyle, A., Grap, M.J., Younger, J. and Thornby, D. (1991) Personality hardiness, ways of coping, social support and burnout in critical care nurses. *Journal of Advanced Nursing*, 16: 850–7.

Bradbury, M. (1996) Representations of 'good' and 'bad' death among deathworkers and the bereaved, in G. Howarth and P.C. Jupp (eds) *Contemporary Issues in the Sociology of Death, Dying and Disposal*. Basingstoke: Macmillan.

British Medical Association (1999) *Withholding and Withdrawing Life-Prolonging Medical Treatment*. London: British Medical Association.

Buckman, R. (1992) *How to Break Bad News: A Guide for Health Professionals*. London: Macmillan.

Bury, M.R. (1986) Social constructionism and the development of medical sociology. *Sociology of Health and Illness*, 8: 137–69.

Calnan, M. and Williams, S. (1992) Images of scientific medicine. *Sociology of Health and Illness*, 14: 233–54.

Calnan, M. and Williams, S. (1994) Lay perceptions of modern medicine and modern medical practice, in I. Robinson (ed.) *The Social Consequences of Life and Death Technology Medicine*. Manchester: Manchester University Press.

Campbell, M.L. and Frank, R.R. (1997) Experience with end of life practice at a university hospital. *Critical Care Medicine*, 25: 197–202.

Cartwright, W. (1996) Killing and letting die: a defensible distinction? *British Medical Bulletin*, 52: 354–61.

Christakis, N.A. and Asch, D.A. (1993) Biases in how physicians choose to withdraw life support. *Lancet*, 343: 642–6.

Cicourel, A.V. (1974) *Cognitive Sociology: Language and Meaning in Social Interaction*. New York: Free Press.

Cicourel, A.V. (1990) The integration of distributed knowledge in collaborative medical diagnosis, in J. Galegher, R.E. Kraut and C. Egido (eds) *Intellectual Teamwork: Social and Technological Foundations of Co-operative Work*. Hillsdale, NJ: Lawrence Erlbaum.

Clark, D. (1998) Originating a movement: Cicely Saunders and the development of St Christopher's Hospice. *Mortality*, 3: 43–63.

Clark, D. and Seymour, J. (1999) *Reflections on Palliative Care: Sociological and Policy Perspectives*. Buckingham: Open University Press.

Clark, J.A., Potter, D.A. and McKinlay, J.B. (1991) Bringing social structure back into clinical decision making. *Social Science and Medicine*, 32: 853–66.

Cook, D.J. (1997) Health professional decision-making in the ICU: a review of the evidence. *New Horizons*, 5: 15–19.

Cooper, M.C. (1993) The intersection of technology and care in the ICU. *Advanced Nursing Science*, 15(3): 23–32.

Cooper, M.C. (1994) Care: antidote for nurses' love-hate relationship with technology. *American Journal of Critical Care*, 3(5): 402–3.

Corley, M.C. (1995) Moral distress of critical care nurses. *American Journal of Critical Care*, 4: 280–5.

Coulter, M.A. (1989) The needs of family members of patients in intensive care units. *Intensive Care Nursing*, 5: 4–10.

Coyne, P. (1996) Developing nurse consultancy in clinical practice. *Nursing Times,* 92: 34–5.

Crane, D. (1975) *The Sanctity of Social Life.* New York: Russell Sage.

Cray, L. (1989) A collaborative project: initiating a family intervention program in a medical intensive care unit. *Focus on Critical Care,* 16: 212–18.

Crosby, D.L. and Rees, G.A.D. (1994) Provision of post-operative care in UK hospitals. *Annals of the Royal College of Surgeons in England,* 75: 14–18.

Cudmore, J. (1996) Do nurses perceive that there is a need for defusing and debriefing following the resuscitation of a patient in the accident and emergency department? *Nursing in Critical Care,* 1: 188–93.

Danis, M. (1998) Improving end-of-life care in the intensive care unit: what's to be learned from outcomes research? *New Horizons,* 6: 110–18.

de Raeve, L. (1996) Dignity and integrity at the end of life. *International Journal of Palliative Nursing,* 2: 71.

Debate of the Age Health and Care Study Group (1999) *The Future of Health and Care of Older People: The Best is Yet to Come.* London: Age Concern.

Degner, L.F. and Beaton, J.I. (1987) *Life and Death Decisions in Health Care.* Cambridge, New York, Philadelphia: Hemisphere.

Department of Health (1989) *Working for Patients.* London: HMSO.

Department of Health (1991) *The Patients' Charter.* London: HMSO.

Department of Health (1996) *Guidelines for Admission to and Discharge from Intensive and High Dependency Care.* London: HMSO.

Dimond, B. (1990) *Legal Aspects of Nursing.* London: Prentice Hall.

Doyal, L. (1995) Advanced directives. *British Medical Journal,* 310: 612–13.

Dracup, K. and Raffin, T. (1989) Withholding and withdrawing ventilation: assessing quality of life. *American Review of Respiratory Disease,* 140: S40–S46.

Dragsted, L. and Qvist, J. (1992) Epidemiology of intensive care. *International Journal of Technological Assessment in Health Care,* 8: 395–407.

Dunnell, K. (1997) *The Health of Adult Britain 1841–1994.* London: Office of National Statistics.

Eisenberg, J.M. (1979) Sociologic influences on decision-making by clinicians. *Annals of Internal Medicine,* 90: 957–64.

Elias, N. (1985) *The Loneliness of the Dying.* Oxford: Blackwell.

Erlan, J.A. and Frost, B. (1991) Nurses perceptions of powerlessness in influencing ethical decisions. *Western Journal of Nursing Research,* 13: 397–407.

Ersser, S. and Tutton, E. (1991) *Primary Nursing in Perspective.* London: Scutari Press.

Faber-Langendoen, K. (1996) A multi-institutional study of care given to patients in hospitals: ethical and practice implications. *Archives Internal Medicine,* 159: 2130–6.

Faber-Langendoen, K. and Bartels, D.M. (1992) The process of forgoing life sustaining treatment in a university hospital: an empirical study. *Critical Care Medicine,* 20: 570–7.

Farrington, A. (1997) Strategies for reducing stress and burnout in nursing. *British Journal of Nursing,* 6: 44–50.

Field, D. (1989) *Nursing the Dying.* London: Tavistock/Routledge.

Field, D. (1994) Palliative medicine and the medicalization of death. *European Journal of Cancer Care,* 3: 58–62.

Field, D. (1996) Awareness and modern dying. *Mortality*, 1: 255–65.

Field, P. (1991) Doing fieldwork in your own culture, in J.M. Morse (ed.) *Qualitative Nursing Research: A Contemporary Dialogue*. Newbury Park, CA: Sage.

Firth, S. (1996) The good death: attitudes of British Hindus, in G. Howarth and P.C. Jupp (eds) *Contemporary Issues in the Sociology of Death, Dying and Disposal*. Basingstoke: Macmillan.

Fisher, S. (1984) Doctor–patient communication: a social and micro political performance. *Sociology of Health and Illness*, 6: 1–29.

Foucault, M. (1976) *The Birth of the Clinic: An Archaeology of Medical Perception*. London: Tavistock.

Fox, N. (1992) *The Social Meaning of Surgery*. Buckingham: Open University Press.

Fox, N. (1993) *Postmodernism, Sociology and Health*. Buckingham: Open University Press.

Fox, N. (1994) Anaesthetists, the discourse on patient fitness and the organization of surgery. *Sociology of Health and Illness*, 16: 1–18.

Fox, R. (1959) *Experiment Perilous: Physicians and Patients Facing the Unknown*. Glencoe, IL: Free Press.

Freidson, E. (1970) *Profession of Medicine: A Study of the Sociology of Applied Knowledge*. New York: Dodd, Mead and Company.

Fulbrook, P., Allan, D., Carroll, S. and Dawson, D. (1999a) On the receiving end: experiences of being a relative in critical care. Part 1. *Nursing in Critical Care*, 4: 138–45.

Fulbrook, P., Buckley, P., Mills, G. and Smith, G. (1999b) On the receiving end: experiences of being a relative in critical care. Part 2. *Nursing in Critical Care*, 4: 179–85.

Fulbrook, P., Creasey, J., Langford, D. and Manley, K. (1999c) On the receiving end: experiences of being a relative in critical care. Part 3. *Nursing in Critical Care*, 4: 222–30.

Furukawa, M.M. (1996) Meeting the needs of the dying patient's family. *Critical Care Nurse*, 16: 51–7.

Gelder, M.S. (1995) Life and death decisions in the Intensive Care Unit. *Cancer Supplement*, 76: 2171–5.

Giddens, A. (1990) *The Consequences of Modernity*. Cambridge: Polity Press.

Giddens, A. (1991) *Modernity and Self-identity: Self and Society in the Late Modern Age*. Cambridge: Polity Press.

Gilbertson, A.A. (1995) Before intensive therapy? *Journal of the Royal Society of Medicine*, 88: 459p–463p.

Glaser, B.G. and Strauss, A. (1965) *Awareness of Dying*. Chicago: Aldine.

Goffman, E. (1968) *Stigma: Notes on the Management of Spoiled Identity*. Harmondsworth: Penguin.

Goffman, E. (1974) *Frame Analysis*. New York: Harper Row.

Goldhill, D.R. and Sumner, A. (1998) Outcome of intensive care patients in a group of British intensive care units. *Critical Care Medicine*, 26: 1337–45.

Goldhill, D.R., Worthington, L.M. and Mulcahy, A.J. (1998) (Letter) Quality of care before admission to intensive care. *British Medical Journal*, 318: 195.

Gordon, D. (1988) Clinical science and clinical expertise: changing boundaries between art and science in medicine, in M. Lock and D. Gordon (eds) *Biomedicine Examined*. Dordrecht: Kluwer Academic.

Gordon, M. and Singer, P.A. (1995) Decisions and care at the end of life. *Lancet*, 346: 163–6.

Griffin, J. (1991) *Dying with Dignity*. London: Office of Health Economics.

Griffiths, L. (1997) Accomplishing team: teamwork and categorization in two community mental health teams. *Sociological Review*, 45: 59–74.

Gunning, K. and Rowan, K. (1999) ABC of intensive care: outcome data and scoring systems. *British Medical Journal*, 319: 241–4.

Hale, C. (1995) Case management and managed care. *Nursing Standard*, 9: 33–5.

Hall, B. and Hall, D.A. (1994) Learning from the experience of loss: people bereaved during intensive care. *Intensive and Critical Care Nursing*, 10: 265–70.

Hall-Smith, J., Ball, C. and Coakley, J. (1997) Follow-up services and the development of a clinical nurse specialist in intensive care. *Intensive & Critical Care Nursing*, 13: 243–8.

Hancock, C. (1992) *Named Nurse*. Open letter to Royal College of Nursing Members. London: RCN.

Handy, J. (1991) Stress and contradiction in psychiatric nursing. *Human Relations*, 44: 39–53.

Harvey, J. (1994) Researching major life events. *Studies in Qualitative Methodology*, 4: 137–70.

Harvey, J. (1996) Achieving the indeterminate: accomplishing degrees of certainty in life and death situations. *The Sociological Review*, 44: 78–98.

Harvey, J. (1997) The technological regulation of death: with reference to the technological regulation of birth. *Sociology*, 31: 719–35.

Hennemen, E.A., Lee, J.L. and Cohen, J.L. (1995) Collaboration: a concept analysis. *Journal of Advanced Nursing*, 21: 103–9.

Hilberman, M. (1975) The evolution of intensive care units. *Critical Care Medicine*, 3: 159–65.

Hochschild, A. (1983) *The Managed Heart*. Berkeley, CA: University of California Press.

Hockey, J. (1996) The view from the west: reading the anthropology of non-western death ritual, in G. Howarth and P.C. Jupp (eds) *Contemporary Issues in the Sociology of Death, Dying and Disposal*. Basingstoke: Macmillan.

Holloway, I. and Wheeler, S. (1995) Ethical issues in qualitative nursing research. *Nursing Ethics*, 2: 223–32.

Hopkins, P.D. (1997) Why does removing machines count as 'passive' euthanasia? *Hastings' Center Report*, 27: 29–37.

House of Lords' Select Committee on Medical Ethics (1994) *Report of the Committee on Medical Ethics*. (1993–4) (HL 21-I). London: HMSO.

Howse, K. (1998) Health care rationing, non-treatment and euthanasia: ethical dilemmas. In M. Bernard and J. Phillips (eds) *The Social Policy of Old Age: Moving into the 21st Century*. London: Centre for Policy on Ageing.

Hoyt, J.W. (1995) Medical futility. *Critical Care Medicine*, 23: 621–2.

Hughes, D. (1988) When nurse knows best: some aspects of nurse/doctor interaction in a casualty department. *Sociology of Health and Illness*, 19: 1–22.

Hughes, D. and Griffiths, L. (1997) 'Ruling in' and 'ruling out': two approaches to the micro rationing of health care. *Social Science and Medicine*, 44: 589–99.

Hunter, A.R. (1967) Intensive care as a specialty. *Lancet*, 1: 1151–3.

Illich, I. (1976) *Limits to Medicine/Medical Nemesis: The Expropriation of Health*. London: Penguin Books.

Jackson, I. (1996) Critical care nurses' perceptions of a bereavement follow up service. *Intensive and Critical Care Nursing*, 12: 2–11.

James, N. (1989) Emotional labour: skill and work in the social regulation of feelings. *Sociological Review*, 37: 15–42.

James, N. (1992) Care = organization + physical labour + emotional labour. *Sociology of Health and Illness*, 14: 488–509.

James, V. and Field, D. (1996) Who has the power? Some problems and issues affecting the nursing care of dying patients. *European Journal of Cancer Care*, 5: 73–80.

Jennett, B. (1984) Inappropriate use of intensive care. *British Medical Journal*, 289: 1709–10.

Jennett, B. (1994) Treatment of critical illness in the elderly. *Hastings' Center Report*, 24: 21–2.

Johnson, K. (1993) A moral dilemma: killing and letting die. *British Journal of Nursing*, 2: 635–40.

Johnston, S.C. and Pfeifer, M.P. (1998) Patient and physician roles in end-of-life decision making. End-of-Life study Group. *Journal of General Internal Medicine*, 13: 43–5.

Jones, C., Hussey, R.M. and Griffiths, R.D. (1991) Social support in the ICU? *British Journal of Intensive Care*, 1: 67–9.

Karlawish, J.H.T. (1996) Shared decision making in critical care: a clinical reality and an ethical necessity. *American Journal of Critical Care*, 5: 391–6.

Kastenbaum, R. (1969) Psychological death, in L. Pearson (ed.) *Dying and Death*. Cleveland, OH: Western Reserve University Press.

Kastenbaum, R. and Aisenberg, R. (1972) *The Psychology of Death*. New York: Springer.

Katz, P. (1985) How surgeons make decisions, in R.A. Hahn and A.D. Gaines (eds) *Physicians of Western Medicine: Anthropological Approaches to Theory and Practice*. Dordrecht: Reidel.

Kaufman, S.R. (1998) Intensive care, old age, and the problem of death in America. *The Gerontologist*, 38: 715–25.

Kellehear, A. (1990) *Dying of Cancer: The Final Year of Life*. Melbourne: Harwood Academic Publishers.

Kelner, M. (1995) Activists and delegators: elderly patients' preferences about control at the end of life. *Social Science and Medicine*, 41: 537–45.

Kissane, D.W., Bloch, S., Onghena, P., *et al.* (1996) The Melbourne Family Grief Study 1. Psychosocial morbidity and grief in bereaved families. *American Journal of Psychiatry*, 153(3): 659–66.

Knafl, K. and Burkett, G. (1975) Professional socialization in a surgical specialty: acquiring medical judgement. *Social Science and Medicine*, 9: 394–404.

Knaus, W.A., Draper, E.A., Wagner, D.P. and Zimmerman, J.E. (1985) APACHE II: a severity of disease classification system. *Critical Care Medicine*, 13: 18–29.

Knaus, W.A., Wagner, D.P., Draper, E.A. *et al.* (1991) The APACHE III prognostic system. Risk prediction of hospital mortality for critically ill hospitalized adults. *Chest*, 100: 1619–36.

Koch, K.A., Rodeffer, H.D. and Wears, R.L. (1994) Changing patterns of terminal care management in an intensive care unit. *Critical Care Medicine*, 22: 233–43.

Kübler-Ross, E. (1970) *On Death and Dying*. London: Tavistock.

Kübler-Ross, E. (1975) *Death: The Final Stage of Growth*. Englewood Cliffs, NJ: Prentice Hall.

Law Commission for England and Wales (1995) *Mental Incapacity* (Report no. 231). London: HMSO.

Lawler, J. (1991) *Behind the Screens: Nursing, Somology, and the Problem of the Body*. London: Churchill-Livingstone.

Le Fanu, J. (1999) *The Rise and Fall of Modern Medicine*. London: Little Brown and Company.

Leske, J. (1992) Impact of critical injury as described by a spouse: a retrospective case study. *Clinical Nursing Research*, 1: 385–401.

Lindemann, E. (1944) Symptomatology and the management of acute grief. *American Journal of Psychiatry*, 101: 141–8.

Lo, B. (1995) Improving care near the end of life. Why is it so hard? *Journal of the American Medical Association*, 274: 1634–6.

Lofland, L. (1978) *The Craft of Dying*. Beverley Hills, CA: Sage.

Lupton, D. (1994) *Medicine as Culture: Illness, Disease and the Body in Western Societies*. London: Sage.

Lupton, D. (1995) Perspectives on power, communication and the medical encounter: implications for nursing theory and practice. *Nursing Inquiry*, 2: 157–63.

Lupton, D. (1996) Your life in their hands: trust in the medical encounter, in V. James and J. Gabe (eds) *Health and the Sociology of Emotions*. Oxford: Blackwell.

Lupton, D. (1997) Foucault and the medicalization critique, in A.R. Peterson and R. Bunton (eds) *Foucault, Health and Medicine*. New York: Routledge.

Lynaugh, J.E. and Fairman, J. (1992) New nurses, new spaces: a preview of the AACN history study. *American Journal of Critical Care*, 1: 19–24.

Mackay, L. (1993) *Conflicts in Care: Medicine and Nursing*. London: Chapman and Hall.

Manley, K. (1988) The needs and support of relatives. *Nursing*, 3: 19–22.

Manthey, M. (1992) *The Practice of Primary Nursing*. London: King's Fund Centre.

May, C. (1991) Affective neutrality and the involvement in nurse patient relationships-perceptions of appropriate behaviour among nurses in acute medical and surgical wards. *Journal of Advanced Nursing*, 16: 552–8.

May, C. (1992a) Individual care? Power and subjectivity in therapeutic relationships. *Sociology*, 26: 589–602.

May, C. (1992b) Nursing work, nurses' knowledge and the subjectification of the patient. *Sociology of Health and Illness*, 14: 472–87.

McFall, L. (1987) Integrity. *Ethics*, 98: 5–20.

McIntosh, J. (1977) *Communication and Awareness in a Cancer Ward*. London: Croom Helm.

McMahon, J. (1993) Killing, letting die and withdrawing aid. *Ethics*, 103: 250–79.

McNamara, B., Waddell, C. and Colvin, M. (1994) The institutionalization of the good death. *Social Science and Medicine*, 39: 1501–8.

McQuillan, P., Pilkington, S., Allan, A., *et al.* (1998) Confidential inquiry into the quality of care before admission to intensive care. *British Medical Journal,* 316: 1853–63.

Menzies, I. (1970) *The Functioning of Social Systems as a Defence Against Anxiety.* (Reprint of Tavistock Pamphlet 3) London: Tavistock Institute.

Metcalfe, M.A. and McPherson, K. (1994) *Study of Provision of Intensive Care in England.* London: London School of Hygiene and Tropical Medicine.

Metcalfe, M.A., Slogett, A. and McPherson, K. (1997) Mortality among appropriately referred patients refused admission to intensive care units. *Lancet,* 350: 7–11.

Miller, F.G. and Brody, H. (1995) Professional integrity and physician-assisted death. *Hastings' Center Report,* 25: 8–17.

Millman, M. (1976) *The Unkindest Cut: Life in the Backrooms of Medicine.* New York: William Morrow.

Mitchell, J.C. (1983) Case and situation analysis. *Sociological Review,* 31: 187–211.

Moller, D.W. (1990) *On Death without Dignity: the Human Impact of Technological Dying.* Amityville, NY: Baywood.

Moller, D.W. (1996) *Confronting Death: Values, Institutions and Human Mortality.* New York, Oxford: Oxford University Press.

Molter, N.C. (1979) Needs of relatives of critically ill patients: a descriptive study. *Heart Lung,* 8: 332–9.

Moskowitz, E.H. and Nelson J.L. (1995) The best laid plans. *Hastings' Center Report (Supplement),* November-December: 53–5.

Muller, J.H. and Koenig, B.A. (1988) On the boundary of life and death: the definition of dying by medical residents, in M. Lock and D.R. Gordon (eds) *Biomedicine Examined.* Dordrecht: Kluwer.

Nelson, H.L. and Nelson, J.L. (1995) *The Patient in the Family: An Ethics of Medicine and Families.* London: Routledge.

Nicholson, M. and McLaughlin, C. (1987) Social constructionism and medical sociology: a reply to M.R. Bury. *Sociology of Health and Illness,* 9: 207–26.

Nicholson, M. and McLanghlin, C. (1988) Social constructionism and medical sociology: a study of the vascular theory of multiple sclerosis. *Sociology of Health and Illness,* 10: 234–61.

Nolan, M. (1995) Towards an ethos of interdisciplinary practice. *British Medical Journal,* 311: 305–7.

Pabst-Battin, M. (1994) *The Least Worst Death. Essays in Bioethics on the End of Life.* Oxford: Oxford University Press.

Pappas, D.M. (1996) Recent historical perspectives regarding medical euthanasia and physician assisted suicide. *British Medical Bulletin,* 52: 386–93.

Parrillo, J.E. (1995) A silver anniversary for the Society of Critical Care Medicine – visions of the past and future: the presidential address from the 24th Educational and Scientific Symposium of the Society of Critical Care Medicine (Editorial). *Critical Care Medicine,* 23: 607–12.

Paris, J.J. and Reardon, F.E. (1991) An ethical and legal analysis of problems in critical care medicine, in J.M. Rippe, R.S. Irwin, J.S.A. Alpert, *et al.* (eds) *Intensive Care Medicine.* Boston: Little Brown and Company.

Payne, S.A., Langley-Evans, A. and Hillier, R. (1996) Perceptions of a 'good' death: a comparative study of the views of hospice staff and patients. *Palliative Medicine,* 10: 307–12.

Pearson, A. (1988) Primary nursing, in A. Pearson (ed.) *Primary Nursing: Nursing in the Burford and Oxford Nursing Development Units*. London: Chapman and Hall.

Perakyla, A. (1991) Hope work in the care of seriously ill patients. *Qualitative Health Research*, 1: 407–33.

Peterson, M. (1988) The norms and values held by 3 groups of nurses concerning psychosocial practice. *International Journal of Nursing Studies*, 25: 85–103.

Petryshen, P.R. and Petryshen, P.M. (1992) The case management model: an innovative approach to the delivery of patient care. *Journal of Advanced Nursing*, 17: 1188–94.

Pijnenborg, L., van der Maas, P.J., Kardaun, J.W. *et al.* (1995) Withdrawal or withholding of treatment at the end of life. Results of a nationwide study. *Archives of Internal Medicine*, 155: 286–92.

Poses, M., Bekes, C., Copare, F., *et al.* (1989) The answer to 'What are my chances, Doctor?' depends on who is asked: prognostic disagreement and inaccuracy for critically ill patients. *Critical Care Medicine*, 17: 827–33.

Principal Investigators for the SUPPORT Project (1995) A controlled trial to improve care for seriously ill hospitalized patients: the study to understand prognoses and preferences for outcomes and risks of treatment (SUPPORT). *Journal of the American Medical Association*, 174: 1591–8.

Quint, J.C. (1967) *The Nurse and the Dying Patient*. New York: Macmillan.

Quint-Benoliel, J.C. (1977) Nurses and the human experience of dying, in H. Feifel (ed.) *New Meanings of Death*. New York: McGraw-Hill.

Rachels, J. (1975) Active and passive euthanasia. *New England Medical Journal*, 292: 78–80.

Randall, F. and Downie, R.S. (1996) *Palliative Care Ethics: a Good Companion*. Oxford: Oxford University Press.

Reiser, S.J. (1992) The intensive care unit. The unfolding and ambiguities of survival therapy. *International Journal of Technology Assessment in Health Care*, 8: 382–94.

Ridley, S., Biggam, M. and Stone, P. (1990) A cost-benefit analysis of intensive therapy. *Anaesthesia*, 48: 14–19.

Rier, D.A. (2000) The missing voice of the critically ill: a medical sociologist's first person account. *Sociology of Health and Illness*, 22: 68–93.

Ritter, J., Fralic, M.F., Tonges, M.C., *et al.* (1992) Redesigned nursing practice: a case management model for critical care. *Nursing Clinics of North America*, 27: 119–28.

Rodney, P. (1988) Moral distress in critical care nursing. *Canadian Critical Care Nursing Journal*, 5: 9–11.

Roth, M. (1996) Euthanasia and related ethical issues in dementias of later life with special reference to Alzheimer's disease. *British Medical Bulletin*, 52: 263–79.

Salvage, J. (1990) The theory and practice of the 'new nursing'. *Nursing Times Occasional Paper*, 86: 42–5.

Salvage, J. (1995) What's happening to nursing: the traditional division of labour between doctors and nurses is changing. *British Medical Journal*, 311: 274–5.

Saunders, J.M. and Valente, S.M. (1994) Nurse's grief. *Cancer Nursing*, 17: 318–25.

Savage, J. (1995) *Nursing Intimacy: An Ethnographic Approach to Nurse Patient Interaction*. London: Scutari Press.

Schapira, D.V., Studnicki, J., Bradham, D.D., *et al.* (1993) Intensive care, survival and expense of treating critically ill cancer patients. *Journal of the American Medical Association*, 269: 783–6.

Schecter, S., Capalbo, C.J., Bowen, J.R. and Perry, T. (1998) On the development of the surgical intensive care unit: the Rhode Island Experience. *Medicine and Health Rhode Island*, 81(10): 318–20.

Schneiderman, L.J., Jecker, N.S. and Jonsen, A.R. (1990) Medical futility: its meaning and ethical implications. *Annals of Internal Medicine*, 112: 949–54.

Scholes, J., Furlong, S. and Vaughan, B. (1999) New roles in practice: charting the typologies of role innovation. *Nursing in Critical Care*, 4: 268–75.

Schön, D. (1983) *The Reflective Practitioner*. New York: Basic Books.

Schutz, A. (1964) *Collected Papers: Studies in Social Theory*. The Hague: Nijhoff.

Seale, C. (1995a) Dying alone. *Sociology of Health and Illness*, 17: 377–91.

Seale, C. (1995b) Heroic death. *Sociology*, 29: 597–613.

Seale, C. and Cartwright, A. (1994) *The Year before Death*. Aldershot: Avebury.

Searle, J.F. (1996) Euthanasia: the intensive care unit. *British Medical Bulletin*, 52: 289–95.

Silverman, D. (1987) *Communication and Medical Practice: Social Relations in the Clinic*. London: Sage.

Simpson, S.H. (1994) A study into the use and effects of do not resuscitate orders in the intensive care units of two teaching hospitals. *Intensive and Critical Care Nursing*, 10: 12–22.

Simpson, S.H. (1997) Reconnecting: the experiences of nurses caring for hopelessly ill patients in intensive care. *Intensive and Critical Care Nursing*, 13: 189–97.

Singer, P. (1994) *Rethinking Life and Death: The Collapse of Our Traditional Ethics*. Oxford: Oxford University Press.

Slomka, J. (1992) The negotiation of death: clinical decision making at the end of life. *Social Science and Medicine*, 35: 251–9.

Small, N. (1997) Death and difference, in D. Field, J. Hockey and N. Small (eds) *Death, Gender and Ethnicity*. London: Routledge.

Smedira, N.G., Evans, B.H., Grais, L.S., *et al.* (1990) Withholding and withdrawal of life support from the critically ill. *New England Journal of Medicine*, 322: 309–15.

Smith, P. (1992) *The Emotional Labour of Nursing*. Basingstoke: Macmillan.

Stein, L. (1967) The doctor-nurse game. *Archives of General Psychiatry*, 16: 699–703.

Stein, L., Watts, D. and Howell, T. (1990) The doctor-nurse game revisited. *New England Journal of Medicine*, 322: 546–9.

Strauss, A. (1979) *Negotiations, Varieties, Context, Processes and Social Order*. San Francisco, CA: Jossey Bass.

Strauss, A.L., Fagerhaugh, S., Suczek, B. and Wiener, C. (1985) *The Social Organization of Medical Work*. Chicago: University of Chicago Press.

Strong, P. (1979) *The Ceremonial Order of the Clinic: Patient, Doctors and Medical Bureaucracies*. London: Routledge Kegan Paul.

Stroud, R. (1997) The effects of technology on relatives in critical care environments. *Nursing in Critical Care*, 2: 272–5.

Sudnow, D. (1967) *Passing On: The Social Organization of Dying*. Englewood Cliffs, NJ: Prentice Hall.

Svensson, R. (1996) The interplay between doctors and nurses: a negotiated order perspective. *Sociology of Health and Illness*, 18: 379–98.

Swanson, K. (1991) Empirical development of a middle range theory of caring. *Nursing Research*, 40: 161–6.

Tahan, H.A. (1999) Clarifying case management: what is in a label? *Lippincott's Case Management*, 4(6): 268–78.

Tanner, C.A., Benner, P. and Chelsa, C. (1993) The phenomenology of knowing the patient. *IMAGE: Journal of Nursing Scholarship*, 25: 273–80.

Task Force on Ethics of the Society of Critical Care Medicine (1990) Consensus report on the ethics of foregoing life-sustaining treatments in the critically ill. *Critical Care Medicine*, 18: 1435–9.

Teres, D. (1993) Trends from the United States with end of life decisions in the intensive care unit. *Intensive Care Medicine*, 19: 316–22.

Thompson, F.F. and Singer, M. (1995) High dependency units in the UK: variable size, variable character, few in number. *Postgraduate Medical Journal*, 71: 217–22.

Tilden, V., Tolle, S., *et al.* (1995) Decisions about life sustaining treatment: impact of physicians' behaviour on the family. *Archives of Internal Medicine*, 155: 633–8.

Timmermans, S. (1998) Resuscitation technology in the emergency department: towards a dignified death. *Sociology of Health and Illness*, 20: 144–67.

Timmermans, S. (1999) *Sudden Death and the Myth of CPR*. Philadelphia, PA: Temple University Press.

Turner, B.S. (1984) *The Body and Society: Explorations in Social Theory*. London: Basil Blackwell.

Turner, B.S. (1996) *The Body and Society*. London: Sage.

Usher, K. and Arthur, D. (1998) Process consent: a model for enhancing informed consent in mental health nursing. *Journal of Advanced Nursing*, 27: 692–7.

Walby, S. and Greenwell, J. (1994) *Medicine and Nursing: Professions in a Changing Health Service*. London: Sage.

Walters, A.J. (1994a) The comforting role in critical care nursing practice: a phenomenological interpretation. *International Journal of Nursing Studies*, 31(6): 607–16.

Walters, A.J. (1994b) An interpretative study of the clinical practice of critical care nurses. *Contemporary Nurse*, 3(1): 21–5.

Walters, A.J. (1995) Technology and the life world of critical care nursing. *Journal of Advanced Nursing*, 22: 338–46.

Wanzer, S.H., Adelstein, J. and Cranford, R. (1984) The physician's responsibility towards hopelessly ill patients. *New England Journal of Medicine*, 310: 955–99.

Wilkinson, P. (1995) A qualitative study to establish the self-perceived needs of family members of patients in the general intensive care unit. *Intensive and Critical Care Nursing*, 11: 77–85.

Wilkinson, S. (1991) Factors which influence how nurses communicate with cancer patients. *Journal of Advanced Nursing*, 16: 667–88.

Williams, R. (1990) *A Protestant Legacy: Attitudes to Death and Dying among Older Aberdonians*. Oxford: Clarendon Press.

Williams, S.J. and Calnan, M. (1996) The 'limits' of medicalization? Modern medicine and the lay populace in 'late' modernity. *Social Science and Medicine*, 42: 1609–20.

Winter, B. and Cohen, S. (1999) ABC of intensive care: withdrawal of treatment. *British Medical Journal*, 319: 306–8.

Wright, P. and Treacher, A. (eds) (1982) *Biomedicine Examined*. Dordrecht: Kluwer.

Wright, S. (1990) *My Patient – My Nurse: The Practice of Primary Nursing*. London: Scutari Press.

Wright, S. (1992) Modelling excellence: the role of the consultant nurse, in T. Butterworth and J. Faugier (eds) *Clinical Supervision and Mentorship in Nursing*. London: Chapman.

Wright, S., Bowkett, J. and Bray, K. (1996) The communication gap in the ICU: a possible solution. *Nursing in Critical Care*, 1: 241–4.

Yarling, R.R. and McElmurry, B.J. (1986) The moral foundation of nursing. *Advances in Nursing Science*, 8: 63–73.

Yeoman, P. and Sleator, A. (1995) *Intensive Care. Inside an Intensive Care Unit*. London: Boxtree Ltd.

Yin, R.K. (1984) *Case Study Research: Design and Methods*. Beverley Hills and London: Sage.

Youll, J.W. (1989) The bridge beyond: strengthening nursing practice in attitudes towards death, dying, and the terminally ill, and helping the spouses of critically ill patients. *Intensive Care Nursing*, 5: 88–94.

Young, M. and Cullen, L. (1996) *A Good Death: Conversations with East Londoners*. London: Routledge.

Zussman, R. (1992) *Intensive Care: Medical Ethics and the Medical Profession*. Chicago, IL: University of Chicago Press.

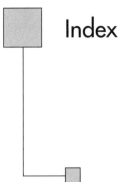

Index

REFLECTIONS ON PALLIATIVE CARE

David Clark and Jane Seymour

Palliative care seems set to continue its rapid development into the early years of the twenty-first century. From its origins in the modern hospice movement, the new multidisciplinary specialty of palliative care has expanded into a variety of settings. Palliative care services are now being provided in the home, in hospital and in nursing homes. There are moves to extend palliative care beyond its traditional constituency of people with cancer. Efforts are being made to provide a wide range of palliative therapies to patients at an early stage of their disease progression. The evidence-base of palliative care is growing, with more research, evaluation and audit, along with specialist programmes of education. Palliative care appears to be coming of age.

On the other hand numbers of challenges still exist. Much service development has been unplanned and unregulated. Palliative care providers must continue to adapt to changing patterns of commissioning and funding services. The voluntary hospice movement may feel its values threatened by a new professionalism and policies which require its greater integration within mainstream services. There are concerns about the re-medicalization of palliative care, about how an evidence-based approach to practice can be developed, and about the extent to which its methods are transferring across diseases and settings.

Beyond these preoccupations lie wider societal issues about the organization of death and dying in late modern culture. To what extent have notions of death as a contemporary taboo been superseded? How can we characterize the nature of suffering? What factors are involved in the debate surrounding end of life care ethics and euthanasia?

David Clark and Jane Seymour, drawing on a wide range of sources, as well as their own empirical studies, offer a set of reflections on the development of palliative care and its place within a wider social context. Their book will be essential reading to any practitioner, policy maker, teacher or student involved in palliative care or concerned about death, dying and life-limiting illness.

Contents
Introduction – Part 1: Death in society – The social meaning of death and suffering – Ageing, dying and grieving – The ethics of dying – Part II: The philosophy and practice of palliative care – History and development – Definitions, components, meanings – Routinization and medicalization – Part III: Policy issues – Policy development and palliative care – The delivery of palliative care services – Part IV: Conclusion – The future for palliative care – References – Index.

224pp   0 335 19454 0 (Paperback)   0 335 19455 9 (Hardback)

RESEARCHING PALLIATIVE CARE

David Field, David Clark, Jessica Corner and Carol Davis (eds)

This book is an essential resource for the improvement of research skills among researchers in palliative care.

- It identifies key methods in palliative care research.
- Provides accessible examples and discussions of practical, methodological and ethical issues.
- Presents examples of good research practice.
- Provides a wide-ranging coverage of the area.

Researching Palliative Care has been designed as a resource for those directly involved in the delivery of palliative care who wish to pursue research but who have little or no formal training for, or experience of, conducting research. It is also intended as a resource for students on the increasing number of specialist palliative care courses, post-qualification short courses and taught Masters courses for health professionals which have 'health research skills' as important or central elements within their programmes. Although there are many general texts on research methods, there are very few which specifically address research issues in palliative care. This book seeks to fill that gap in the literature. It covers the range of research methods that can be appropriately used for research in palliative care by bringing together a selection from the best articles in the field.

Contents

208pp   0 335 20436 8 (Paperback)   0 335 20437 6 (Hardback)

ON BEREAVEMENT
THE CULTURE OF GRIEF

Tony Walter

Insightful and refreshing.

Professor Dennis Klass, Webster University
St Louis, USA

A tour de force.

Dr Colin Murray Parkes, OBE, MD, FRCPsych,
President of CRUSE

Some societies and some individuals find a place for their dead, others leave them behind. In recent years, researchers, professionals and bereaved people themselves have struggled with this. Should the bond with the dead be continued or broken? What is clear is that the grieving individual is not left in a social vacuum but has to struggle with expectations from self, family, friends, professionals and academic theorists.

This ground-breaking book looks at the social position of the bereaved. They find themselves caught between the living and the dead, sometimes searching for guidelines in a de-ritualized society that has few to offer, sometimes finding their grief inappropriately pathologized and policed. At its best, bereavement care offers reassurance, validation and freedom to talk where the client has previously encountered judgmentalism.

In this unique book, Tony Walter applies sociological insights to one of the most personal of human situations. *On Bereavement* is aimed at students on medical, nursing, counselling and social work courses that include bereavement as a topic. It will also appeal to sociology students with an interest in death, dying and mortality.

Contents

Introduction – Part I: Living with the dead – Other places, other times – War, peace and the dead: twentieth-century popular culture – Private bonds – Public bonds: the dead in everyday conversation – The last chapter – Theories – Part II: Policing grief – Guidelines for grief: historical background – Popular guidelines: the English case – Expert guidelines: clinical lore – Vive la différence? The politics of gender – Bereavement care – Conclusion: integration, regulation and postmodernism – References – Index.

256pp   0 335 20080 X (Paperback)   0 335 20081 8 (Hardback)

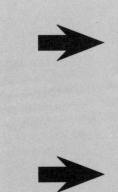
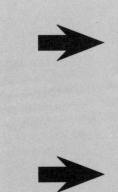